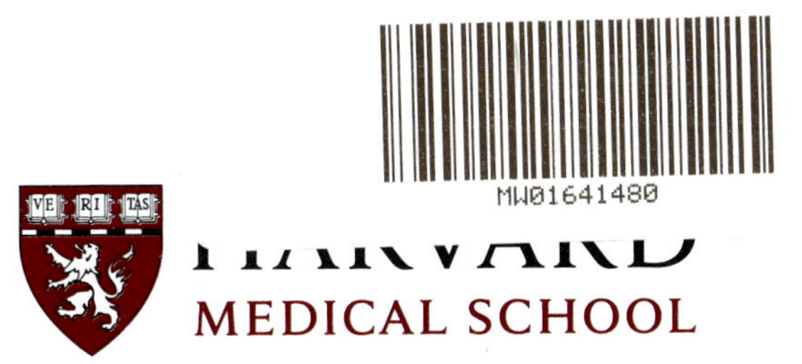

2022 *Annual Report on*
PROSTATE DISEASES

Covering advances in the diagnosis and treatment of prostate cancer, benign prostatic hyperplasia, erectile dysfunction, prostatitis, and related conditions

Published by Harvard Medical School, 4 Blackfan Circle, 4th Floor, Boston, MA 02115

Permissions
Harvard Health Publishing
4 Blackfan Circle, 4th Floor, Boston, MA 02115
www.health.harvard.edu/permissions
Fax: 617-432-1506

Website
For the latest information and most up-to-date publication list, visit us online at www.health.harvard.edu.

Customer Service
For all subscription questions or problems (rates, subscribing, address changes, billing problems), email HarvardProd@StrategicFulfillment.com, call 877-649-9457 (toll-free), or write to Harvard Health Publishing, P.O. Box 9308, Big Sandy, TX 75755-9308.

Ordering Special Health Reports
Harvard Medical School publishes Special Health Reports on a wide range of topics. To order copies of this or other reports, please see the instructions at the back of this report, or go to our website: www.health.harvard.edu.

Licensing, Bulk Rates, or Corporate Sales
email HHP_licensing@hms.harvard.edu, or visit www.health.harvard.edu/licensing.

ISBN 978-1-935555-03-2

2022 Annual Report on

PROSTATE DISEASES

Contents

The *2022 Annual Report on Prostate Diseases* was initially made possible through the philanthropic support of the Gorman, Greimann, and Hershey families.

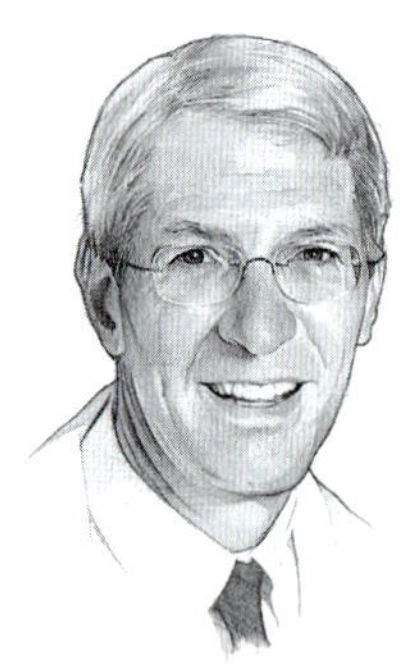

Founding Editor in Chief
Marc B. Garnick, M.D.

A message from the editor in chief

Every year brings remarkable advances in the management and treatment of prostate diseases. With this, the *2022 Annual Report on Prostate Diseases*, we once again bring you up to date on the most significant developments of the past 12 months.

Especially noteworthy is regulatory approval of two imaging agents that reveal where new metastatic prostate tumors are growing in the body. These injectable compounds travel via the bloodstream until they encounter a protein on cancer cell surfaces called prostate-specific membrane antigen (PSMA). They bind to this protein, flagging the cancer cells so they show up on specialized imaging scans, and enabling doctors to find and treat prostate tumors they might otherwise miss. Moreover, by combining PSMA-directed agents with radioactive particles, scientists are developing therapies that target prostate cancer cells with unrivaled precision. In 2021, researchers published clinical trial results showing these experimental therapies extend life span for men with advanced prostate cancer who no longer respond to other treatments.

Genetic testing is another key area where important advances are being made. Scientists in 2021 identified close to 90 additional genetic mutations that increase a man's inherited risk of developing prostate cancer. Clinicians increasingly rely on genetic tests to guide cancer treatments that target specific gene mutations. We provide up-to-date information on the tests being used today and their performance.

Hormonal therapy (also called androgen deprivation therapy) is a mainstay of prostate cancer treatment. We cover the latest news on cardiovascular complications from hormonal therapy, as well as strategies for minimizing them.

In addition, we include a roundtable discussion on exciting developments in treating oligometastatic prostate cancer, which was formerly regarded as incurable, but now in some instances can be considered curable.

Finally, we provide the latest news about benign prostatic hyperplasia, prostatitis, and erectile dysfunction.

We hope you find this edition of the *Annual* to be helpful. We also encourage you to read our 2017 companion publication, *Patient Perspectives on Prostate Diseases*, in which men recount their experiences with many of the treatments described in the *Annual*. We are pleased to be completing our 16th year of publication and look forward to many more years ahead of providing this timely information for our dedicated and expanding readership.

Marc B. Garnick, M.D.
Founding Editor in Chief, *2022 Annual Report on Prostate Diseases*

For more information on the Harvard Special Health Report Patient Perspectives on Prostate Diseases, *go to* www.health.harvard.edu/ps.

A year of progress in prostate research

What made news in 2021

The past year gave rise to many impressive developments in prostate research. Take, for instance, the FDA's approval of new imaging agents, called tracers, used for locating cancer cells that might otherwise evade detection while spreading through the body. These tracers open up new avenues for treating metastatic prostate cancer in its earliest stages, when cures are still within reach.

Hormonal therapies for prostate cancer improve clinical outcomes, but they carry side effects. In 2021, the American Heart Association issued recommendations for managing the cardiovascular complications of these treatments.

Also in 2021, researchers published evidence showing that some men with cancer that progresses (continues to grow) after radiation therapy can be treated with surgical methods that leave portions of the prostate intact, minimizing the potential for urinary dysfunction.

In the following pages, you'll find detailed descriptions of these and other leading stories in prostate research news in 2021, selected by Dr. Marc Garnick, editor in chief of the *Annual*, and Charles Schmidt, editor of the *Annual*. As an added feature this year, we have also asked our editorial board members to comment on a few of the news items.

Axumin PET tracer performs well in real-world settings

Treatments for metastatic prostate cancer are most effective when given at the earliest stages of cancer progression. To visualize small tumors that evade standard imaging tools, doctors use a technology called positron emission tomography (PET). A PET scan relies on injectable tracers that bind to cancer cells. The tracers then show up on the scan, revealing where tumors are located, so that doctors can identify them and develop a suitable treatment plan.

In 2021, researchers published the first study of how the most widely used tracer—fluciclovine F18 (Axumin)—performs in real-world settings. Approved by the FDA in 2016, Axumin is taken up preferentially by cells with high metabolic rates, including cancer cells. Doctors use the tracer to check for metastases in men who have rising prostate-specific antigen (PSA) levels after having surgery or radiation for prostate cancer—a warning that the cancer may be returning.

The investigators reviewed medical records from 165 men with biochemical recurrence who received Axumin PET scans between 2017 and 2019. Seventy of those men had also undergone other types of imaging, including bone scans, computed tomography (CT), and magnetic resonance imaging (MRI). Among all the technologies, Axumin PET was the top performer. None of the men with a negative PET scan

Searching PubMed

You can find any of the studies we've cited in this report by searching online at www.pubmed.gov. For more detailed instructions, see "Searching PubMed in five easy steps," page 120.

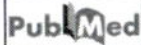

had detectable cancer on other imaging tests. The PET scans also found tumors in nine men for whom CT had not identified cancer, and six men for whom MRI had not identified cancer. Importantly, the PET findings led to treatment of cancers that would otherwise likely have been missed.

Source: Nakamoto R, Harrison C, Song H, et al. The Clinical Utility of ^{18}F-Fluciclovine PET/CT in Biochemically Recurrent Prostate Cancer: An Academic Center Experience Post FDA Approval. *Molecular Imaging and Biology* 2021;23(4):614–23. PMID: 33469884.

FDA approves the first PSMA-targeted PET imaging tracers

Another option for visualizing small, newly forming prostate tumors with PET is to use tracers that bind to proteins on the surface of cancer cells. One such protein is called prostate-specific membrane antigen (PSMA). PSMA exists in normal prostate tissue, but is present in much higher levels in tumors.

The first PSMA-directed tracers have now been approved by the FDA. One of them, known as gallium-68 PSMA-11, identified cancers correctly up to 92% of the time in phase 3 clinical trials (which test how well a new approach works compared with a standard one). To gauge the accuracy of the results, investigators took biopsies of suspected cancer sites flagged by gallium PET imaging and had them checked by a pathologist. However, this tracer is not widely available. The FDA granted approval for its use only at the two academic hospitals where the tracer is manufactured—one based at the University of California, Los Angeles, and the other at the University of California, San Francisco.

The second PSMA-directed tracer, called piflufolastat F18 (Pylarify), was approved in May 2021 for broad distribution. By the fall of 2021, it was already available in parts of the mid-Atlantic and southern regions of the United States and expected to be nationally available by early 2022. Experts anticipate that Pylarify will soon overtake Axumin as the dominant PET tracer for prostate cancer imaging. Men in whom a PSMA scan reveals cancer will also be eligible for a promising experimental treatment called LuPSMA (see next news item).

Sources: FDA. FDA Approves First PSMA-targeted PET Imaging Drug for Men with Prostate Cancer [news release]. Dec. 1, 2020.

FDA. FDA Approves Second PSMA-targeted PET Imaging Drug for Men with Prostate Cancer [news release]. May 27, 2021.

A new treatment for advanced prostate cancer lengthens survival in clinical trials†

Given by intravenous infusion, ^{177}Lu-PSMA-617 (LuPSMA) is like a smart bomb directed at prostate tumors spreading through the body. The drug contains two components: a molecule called PSMA-617, which finds and binds tightly to PSMA, and another called lutetium-177, which delivers radioactive particles that destroy cancer cells.

The first published results with this new treatment came from the TheraP trial, which compared LuPSMA to the chemotherapy drug cabazitaxel (Jevtana) in men with metastatic castration-resistant prostate cancer (mCRPC; see "Prostate cancer terminology," page 38). During this advanced stage of the disease, the cancer no longer responds to drugs that block testosterone, a sex hormone that also fuels prostate

†***Expert commentary from Dr. Anthony L. Zeitman, editorial board member of the Annual:*** *The number of therapeutic options for men with metastatic prostate cancer continues to grow, with an intriguing new agent now being considered by the FDA. This agent is a combination of two molecules, one of which binds to the PSMA found on the surface of prostate cancer cells, and the other of which delivers short-range radioactive particles to kill the cell. This agent, with the rather clumsy name ^{177}Lu-PSMA-617, has previously been shown to seek out metastatic prostate cancer cells and to reduce their activity, and now randomized studies show it can extend life in men with advanced castration-resistant prostate cancer as much as four to five months.*

This finding is good news for men with advanced prostate cancer. But not all patients respond, possibly because the agent has trouble penetrating larger tumors, and also because not all prostate cancer cells have PSMA on their surface. ^{177}Lu-PSMA-617 will likely get FDA approval, and that will be welcome. Even more welcome, however, will be the opportunity to study it in earlier stages of the disease.

tumor growth. Cabazitaxel is given as an alternative treatment, and doctors monitor how well the drug is working by checking a man's PSA level, which rises if the cancer is worsening. Results from the TheraP trial showed that PSA levels fell by half or more in 66% of the LuPSMA-treated men, compared with 37% of the men treated with cabazitaxel.

The next published study—the VISION trial—compared LuPSMA to a standard regimen that did not include cabazitaxel. And again, the men treated with LuPSMA fared better. Cancer progression was delayed by an average of 8.7 months, compared with 3.4 months on the standard therapy, and overall survival was 15.3 months, compared with 11.3 months among patients who did not get the drug.

Now being considered for approval by the FDA, LuPSMA marks a significant development in the treatment of advanced prostate cancer.

Sources: Hofman MS, Emmett L, Sandhu S, et al. [^{177}Lu]Lu-PSMA-617 Versus Cabazitaxel in Patients with Metastatic Castration-Resistant Prostate Cancer (TheraP): A Randomized, Open-Label, Phase 2 Trial. *Lancet* 2021;397(10276):797–804. PMID: 33581798.

Sartor O, de Bono J, Chi KN, et al. Lutetium-177-PSMA-617 for Metastatic Castration-Resistant Prostate Cancer. *New England Journal of Medicine* 2021;385(12):1091–103. PMID: 34161051.

American Heart Association issues statement on cardiovascular risks from hormonal therapy for prostate cancer

Hormonal therapy—also known as androgen deprivation therapy (ADT)—is a cornerstone of prostate cancer treatment. Doctors typically use it for treating newly diagnosed metastatic cancer that is spreading in the body, or cancer that returns after initial treatment with surgery or radiation. But blocking testosterone with hormonal agents can also aggravate symptoms associated with metabolic syndrome. Characterized by increased blood pressure, high blood sugar, excess body fat around the waist, and abnormal cholesterol or triglyceride levels, metabolic syndrome is in turn a risk factor for heart disease and stroke.

The potential for hormonal therapy to worsen existing heart disease is raising concerns. To increase awareness of these potential problems, the American Heart Association (AHA) issued a comprehensive statement in 2021 urging clinicians to monitor heart health closely in men undergoing hormonal therapy, especially if they already have cardiac risk factors or a family history of heart disease.

To protect against cardiometabolic effects from hormonal therapy, the AHA recommended that doctors and patients adhere to the ABCDE strategy:

- **A**ssessment of heart disease risk and taking medication, if needed, to help prevent unwanted clotting
- **B**lood pressure management
- **C**holesterol reduction
- **C**igarette (smoking) cessation
- **D**iet and weight control
- **E**xercise.

The AHA also recommended that men be monitored for signs of metabolic syndrome or uncontrolled cardiovascular risk factors such as high blood pressure.

Source: Okwuosa TM, Morgans A, Rhee JW, et al. Impact of Hormonal Therapies for Treatment of Hormone-Dependent Cancers (Breast and Prostate) on the Cardiovascular System: Effects and Modifications: A Scientific Statement from the American Heart Association. *Circulation: Genomic and Precision Medicine* 2021;14(3):e000082. PMID: 33896190.

Highly anticipated study of cardiovascular risk from different hormonal therapies ends in a draw

Several types of hormonal therapies are used for treating prostate cancer. One class of these drugs, called luteinizing hormone–releasing hormone (LHRH) agonists, triggers an initial surge of testosterone that lasts a few weeks before the hormone's level plummets. Another class of hormonal therapies, gonadotropin-releasing hormone (GnRH) antagonists, suppresses testosterone without the initial surge.

Which of these two drug classes is safer for the heart is an important question. Scientists had hoped that a major international study completed in 2021 would give a clear answer, but it did not. The PRONOUNCE trial, launched in 2016, set out to enroll 900 men with prostate cancer and a history of cardiovascular disease. Study investigators working in 12 countries randomly assigned the men to treatment with either a GnRH antagonist called degarelix (Firmagon)* or an LHRH agonist called leuprolide (Lupron).

**Editor's note:* Dr. Marc Garnick, editor in chief of the Annual, previously served as a consultant to Ferring Pharmaceuticals, the manufacturer of degarelix. He also served as an expert on patent issues related to abiraterone and enzalutamide, both of which are mentioned later in this chapter.*

However, by 2020, only 545 men had enrolled and completed treatment with either therapy. By that time, 15 patients in the degarelix group had suffered a heart attack, stroke, or heart-related death, compared with 11 men in the leuprolide group. Since these numbers were too small to show statistically meaningful differences in cardiac risk between the two drugs, the results from this highly anticipated study were inconclusive. The investigators attributed the enrollment shortfall to changes in the standard of care and the availability of second-generation hormonal therapies that complicated efforts to analyze the data.

Source: Lopes RD, Higano CS, Slovin SF, et al. Cardiovascular Safety of Degarelix Versus Leuprolide in Patients with Prostate Cancer: The Primary Results of the PRONOUNCE Randomized Trial. *Circulation* 2021;144(16):1295–307. PMID: 34459214.

Researchers link hormonal therapies for advanced prostate cancer to higher fall risk

Doctors can also treat advanced prostate cancer with a different class of hormonal therapies, called anti-androgens. Where standard hormonal therapies block testosterone, anti-androgens block one of the hormone's metabolites—a molecule called dihydrotestosterone, which the body manufactures from testosterone. Anti-androgens reduce pain and delay tumor progression. But they have side effects, including nausea, liver problems, and fatigue. A review published in 2021 examined the degree to which anti-androgens may also increase the risk of falls and broken bones.

The investigators focused on three recently approved anti-androgens—apalutamide (Erleada), enzalutamide (Xtandi),* and darolutamide (Nubeqa)—and analyzed nearly a dozen prior studies to see whether any of the drugs posed a greater fall risk than the others. In all, they evaluated 11 studies that involved a total of 11,382 men (average age 72) who had either anti-androgen treatment or some other therapy, whether a placebo or another hormonal therapy that did not involve anti-androgens. All the studies excluded men with history of heart disease or seizures.

According to the results, 8% of men on anti-androgens suffered falls, compared with 5% of men in the control group (who did not receive anti-androgens). Moreover, serious fractures occurred more frequently in men who were taking anti-androgens. Apalutamide had the highest fall risk (12%), followed by enzalutamide (8%) and darolutamide (4%).

Just why anti-androgens boost fall risk isn't known. The drugs may weaken men by decreasing skeletal muscle mass and strength. The take-home message is that fall risk, which is already a significant problem in older men, may be exacerbated by anti-androgen treatment.

Source: Myint ZW, Momo HD, Otto DE, et al. Evaluation of Fall and Fracture Risk Among Men with Prostate Cancer Treated with Androgen Receptor Inhibitors: A Systematic Review and Meta-Analysis. *JAMA Network Open* 2020;3(11):e2025826. PMID: 33201234.

Study finds no cognitive impact from treatment for advanced prostate cancer

Medical or pharmaceutical treatments for cancer can be mentally taxing. Some patients experience a condition known as "chemo fog" that makes it hard for them to focus. But research published in 2021 showed no evidence of cognitive decline among men undergoing drug treatment for mCRPC.

The study enrolled 155 men ages 65 and over, most of whom had at least some postsecondary education. Each was treated with one of four different drugs: docetaxel (Taxotere), which is a type of chemotherapy; enzalutamide* or abiraterone (Zytiga),* which are both hormonal therapies; or radium-223 (Xofigo), a radioactive pharmaceutical that treats cancer in the bones. Three cognitive tests were given both before and after the full course of therapy (ranging from six months with docetaxel or radium-223 to 11 months with enzalutamide or abiraterone). One test required the men to connect a series of dots labeled with 25 numbers in order; another called for connecting a series alternating between numbers and letters; and a third assessed cognitive abilities, including short-term memory, orientation, and language.

Results showed no difference in test scores before and after treatment. Based on those encouraging findings, the researchers concluded that most older men will not experience cognitive decline while being treated for mCRPC, regardless of which therapy they receive.

Source: Alibhai SMH, Breunis H, Feng G, et al. Association of Chemotherapy, Enzalutamide, Abiraterone, and Radium 223 with Cognitive Function in Older Men with Metastatic Castration-Resistant Prostate Cancer. *JAMA Network Open* 2021;4(7):e2114694. PMID: 34213559.

Large genetics study shows Blacks at higher risk of prostate cancer

Black Americans are 50% to 75% more likely to develop prostate cancer and twice as likely to die of the disease as their white counterparts. Several factors contribute to this disproportionate risk, including disparities in the quality of health care. A large study published in 2021 shows that genetic factors also play a part.

The researchers combined genetics data from over 237,000 prostate cancer cases worldwide, including men from European, African, East Asian, and Hispanic populations. Scouring this enormous dataset revealed 86 new heritable genetic variations, each of them independently associated with a greater risk of developing prostate cancer. The team then developed a model to assess how these factors influence prostate cancer risk for different ancestry groups. Findings showed that Blacks inherit about twice the prostate cancer risk on average compared with white populations. By contrast, Asians have the lowest genetic risk of the disease.

Source: Conti DV, Darst BF, Moss LC, et al. Trans-Ancestry Genome-Wide Association Meta-Analysis of Prostate Cancer Identifies New Susceptibility Loci and Informs Genetic Risk Prediction. *Nature Genetics* 2021;53(1):65–75. PMID: 33398198.

Studies find little risk of erectile dysfunction after prostate biopsy†

Men often worry that a prostate biopsy might affect their ability to achieve an erection. Studies investigating that risk have generated mixed results. But a pair of analyses published in 2021 provide some welcome findings: while there is an effect on erectile function in the first weeks after a prostate biopsy, most men regain sexual potency within a few months.

Both analyses assessed how biopsies affect sexual potency as measured by a questionnaire called the International Index of Erectile Function-5 (IIEF-5; see Table 9, page 107). Men with the highest IIEF-5 scores (22 to 25) have little to no loss of potency, while lower scores reflect mild, moderate, or more severe problems.

One of the two analyses—the largest conducted so far—combined high-quality data from 47 published studies involving a total of 9,545 men. According to seven of the studies, IIEF-5 scores dropped 4.6 points on average when measured a month after a biopsy, but were back to baseline or close to baseline when questionnaires were completed again three and six months after the procedure. Importantly, eight of the studies found no significant difference in erectile functioning after a biopsy.

The second analysis, which included data from nine previously published studies, produced similar findings: a month after biopsy, IIEF-5 scores had dropped by approximately 2.2 points, but they returned to baseline within three months on average and remained there at six months.

The studies provide encouraging findings. But investigators pointed out that there isn't enough information to compare the differences between biopsy techniques or predict the effect on erectile function from repeat biopsies.

Sources: Fainberg J, Gaffney CD, Pierce H, et al. Erectile Dysfunction is a Transient Complication of Prostate Biopsy: A Systematic Review and Meta-Analysis. *Journal of Urology* 2021;205(3):664–70. PMID: 33026920.

Mehta A, Kim WC, Aswad KG, et al. Erectile Function Post Prostate Biopsy: A Systematic Review and Meta-Analysis. *Urology* 2021;155:1–8. PMID: 33524434.

†***Expert commentary from Dr. Andrew A. Wagner, editorial board member of the* Annual:** *Prostate biopsy is an anxiety-provoking procedure with a small but significant risk of infection or bleeding. In addition, some men are understandably concerned about the possibility of developing erectile dysfunction (ED) afterward.*

The two studies mentioned here reinforce what we see in clinical practice: that routine prostate biopsies do not contribute to significant long-term ED. The two studies found mild, short-term ED at one month after the procedure, which is likely less worrisome than concerns about blood in the semen or generalized anxiety surrounding the possibility of a cancer diagnosis. These studies do not answer the question, "Do many repeat biopsies accelerate ED over time?" To date, there is only circumstantial evidence that repeat biopsies cause ED. More research is needed. Until then, these two studies absolutely help with our understanding of ED in men after prostate biopsy.

COVID-19 is a risk factor for an enlarged prostate

SARS-CoV-2 (the virus that causes COVID-19) was initially thought to infect only the lungs and upper airways. During the past year, however, researchers found that the virus can also infect other organs, including the prostate. Because SARS-CoV-2 triggers tissue-damaging inflammation in other organs, doctors began questioning whether the virus might aggravate the urinary symptoms caused by an enlarged prostate (a condition called benign prostatic hyperplasia, or BPH).

A 2021 review of 52 published papers suggests that SARS-CoV-2 may damage the prostate and worsen BPH symptoms, although specifically how remains unclear. Scientists are looking at roles for both local inflammation (within the prostate) as well as systemic (bodywide) inflammation originating outside the prostate. The investigators recommend that doctors monitor their older male patients for BPH and associated urinary symptoms during the COVID-19 pandemic.

Source: Haghpana A, Masjedi F, Salehipour M, et al. Is COVID-19 a Risk Factor for Benign Prostatic Hyperplasia and Exacerbation of Its Related Symptoms?: A Systematic Review. *Prostate Cancer and Prostatic Diseases* 2021;Electronic publication ahead of print. PMID: 34007019.

Acupuncture improves symptoms of prostatitis

The symptoms of chronic nonbacterial prostatitis, such as painful urination, can be difficult to treat. Drug therapy helps some men, but not others, and that's led researchers to investigate alternatives that might provide some relief.

One option is acupuncture. This ancient therapy, which involves inserting tiny single-use needles into "acupoints" at various locations in the body and then manipulating them manually or with heat or electrical stimulation, has been shown to reduce prostatitis symptoms. Acupuncture is thought to work in part by promoting the release of the body's own painkilling compounds. And in 2021, Chinese researchers published some of the strongest results yet associating it with improvements in pain, urinary dysfunction, anxiety, depression, and quality of life.

The researchers randomly assigned 440 men with prostatitis to receive 20 sessions of either real acupuncture or a sham procedure over an eight-week period. The sham procedure consisted of inserting needles, but not in traditional acupoints. By the end of the treatment period, 60.6% of men in the acupuncture group were reporting a reduction in symptoms, compared with 36.8% of the men who had the sham procedure, and the benefits were still holding up at week 32.

Source: Sun Y, Liu Y, Liu B, et al. Efficacy of Acupuncture for Chronic Prostatitis / Chronic Pelvic Pain Syndrome: A Randomized Trial. *Annals of Internal Medicine* 2021;174(10):1357–66. PMID: 34399062.

2

An introduction to the prostate gland

The where, what, and why of a male-only gland

How can a gland the size of a walnut that weighs only about an ounce cause so much trouble?

One source of problems relates to the prostate's position in a very crowded place in the body. The prostate is located in front of the rectum (the last part of the colon) and just below the bladder, the hollow organ that holds urine before it is excreted out of the body (see Figure 1, below). Trouble stems from the fact that the prostate wraps around the upper part of the urethra, the slender tube that carries urine from the bladder out of the body through the penis. At birth, a baby boy's prostate gland weighs less than half an ounce, and the gland goes through growth spurts during adolescence and young adulthood. It's normal for the prostate to start growing again when men are in their late 40s and 50s. But when it does, the gland may become so enlarged that it presses on the urethra, preventing urine from flowing freely. That leads to a variety of urinary problems. Other sources of prostate trouble include inflammation and cancer. All of these issues are addressed in detail later in this report.

Figure 1. Locating the prostate gland

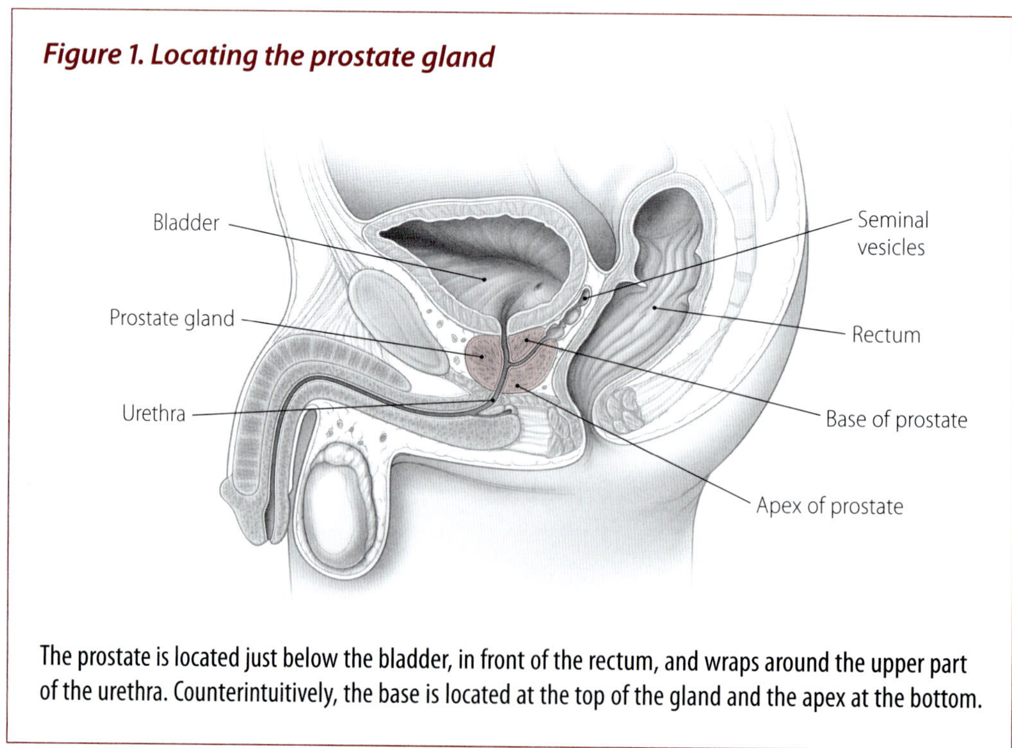

The prostate is located just below the bladder, in front of the rectum, and wraps around the upper part of the urethra. Counterintuitively, the base is located at the top of the gland and the apex at the bottom.

But the prostate performs useful functions as well. While the job of the testicles is to produce sperm, the prostate gland helps supply the semen, the thick, milky fluid that nourishes and protects sperm cells during their travels. The prostate's contribution to semen is alkaline, so it helps sperm survive in the acidic environment of the vagina.

The inside of the gland is made up of an intricate series of ducts lined with cells that produce the prostatic fluid. During ejaculation, the prostate pushes that fluid through those ducts and then into the urethra, where it combines with sperm. Seminal vesicles—slender glands that sit on either side of the prostate—also contribute secretions to semen. By volume, their contribution is actually greater than that of the prostate gland.

The prostate is also tied in to the body's infinitely complex system of hormones. To function properly, it requires adequate amounts of certain hormones. These include testosterone (which is produced by the testicles) as well as other hormones that come from the pituitary gland (which hangs off the base of the brain) and from the adrenal glands (which sit on top of the kidneys).

Although the prostate is sometimes depicted as having a simple round shape, it is actually divided into right and left lobes. It's also tapered at one end. The wider part, called the base, is nestled up next to the bladder; the tip, or apex, is farthest away from the bladder. If the prostate were an arrow, it would be pointing down. If the orientation is front and back, then the front is referred to as the anterior of the gland and the back, the posterior. The area between the base and the apex is referred to as the mid-gland.

These divisions of the gland and the medical terms for them matter when it comes to prostate cancer. Cancers that are located near the base have a propensity to spread to the surrounding tissue, including the seminal vesicles. Cancers in the apex can be difficult to remove surgically, since this location is very close to the muscle that controls urinary continence. Cancer surgery also can threaten two tiny packages of blood vessels and nerves that run along the prostate's surface on each side. Called the neurovascular bundles, they help control a man's ability to have an erection.

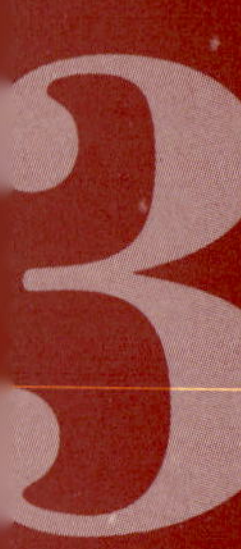

Inflammation of the prostate (prostatitis)

Help for an all-too-common condition

Prostatitis gets little press, but it's a common condition that accounts for nearly two million visits to doctors' offices in the United States each year. Depending on how you define the term, prostatitis (pronounced pros-ta-TIE-tis) affects 9% to 16% of men at some point in their lives. When it comes to age, it's an equal-opportunity disorder: prostatitis affects men of all ages, unlike benign prostatic hyperplasia (BPH) and prostate cancer, which tilt toward an older demographic.

This chapter provides an overview of what leading researchers know about prostatitis, so you can work more effectively with your physician to find a lasting solution.

What is prostatitis?

The *–itis* suffix means inflammation, so prostatitis means inflammation of the prostate. But doctors use the term to refer to a loose assemblage of syndromes characterized by urinary problems such as burning or painful urination, a need to go (urgency), and trouble voiding; difficult or painful ejaculation; and pain in the perineum (the area between the scrotum and the anus) or lower back. Although it causes some of the same symptoms as BPH (see "Lots of LUTS: Symptoms of BPH," page 21) and can occur at the same time, prostatitis is a separate condition.

Some cases of prostatitis are straightforward. They're caused by bacteria that can be easily detected with standard cultures and treated with antibiotics. The symptoms include the classic indications of infection—fever, chills, and muscle pain—as well as urinary problems. But these clear-cut cases are a distinct minority, accounting for just 5% to 10% of cases.

The remaining 90% to 95% of prostatitis cases are harder to get a handle on because of a lack of research and because the causes are complicated and may involve several factors. Often it is difficult, if not impossible, to figure out what triggered a case of chronic (long-term) prostatitis. Among the possible causes are immunological and inflammatory processes that have gone awry. Indeed, mounting evidence suggests the immune system sometimes mistakenly targets the prostate. The resulting autoimmune reactions produce inflammatory compounds that irritate the gland, leading to chronic pain and inflammation. (For references, see "Inflammation and prostatitis," above left.) Other potential causes include bacterial or fungal infections that standard cultures don't detect. Genomic testing of urine has recently reinforced this idea by revealing fragments of bacterial DNA in some men with longstanding prostatitis who experienced a reduction in symptoms after taking antibiotics. (For references, see "Infections and prostatitis," at left.)

Inflammation and prostatitis

Breser ML, Salazar FC, Rivero VE, et al. Immunological Mechanisms Underlying Chronic Pelvic Pain and Prostate Inflammation in Chronic Pelvic Pain Syndrome. *Frontiers in Immunology* 2017;8:898. PMID: 28824626.

Nickel JC, Freedland SJ, Castro-Santamaria R, et al. Chronic Prostate Inflammation Predicts Symptom Progression in Patients with Chronic Prostatitis/Chronic Pelvic Pain. *Journal of Urology* 2017;198(1):122–28. PMID: 28089730.

Infections and prostatitis

Cansizoglu MF, Tamer YT, Farid M, et al. Rapid Ultrasensitive Detection Platform for Antimicrobial Susceptibility Testing. *PLOS Biology* 2019;17(5):e3000291. PMID: 31145726.

Murphy SF, Anker JF, Mazur DJ, et al. Role of Gram-Positive Bacteria in Chronic Pelvic Pain Syndrome (CPPS). *Prostate* 2019;79(2):160–67. PMID: 30242864.

Symptoms may also be triggered by certain compounds in spicy foods, coffee, and alcoholic beverages that irritate the urinary tract. In this case, simply avoiding these foods and drinks will help relieve symptoms. (For reference, see "Diet and prostatitis," at right.)

Another complicating piece of the puzzle is that chronic prostatitis can be accompanied by psychological problems (such as depression, stress, and anxiety). In fact, a 2017 study reported that the presence of accompanying psychological stressors predicts low rates of improvement in prostatitis symptoms over the course of a year. (For references, see "Psychological stress and prostatitis," at right.)

Similarly, another study published in 2017 found that prostatitis often accompanies other chronic pain conditions that might not have an obvious source, such as fibromyalgia, chronic fatigue syndrome, and headaches. These findings suggest that for some patients, holistic treatment strategies that also focus on their ability to cope with pain may be especially promising. Supporting this theory, researchers reported in 2018 that some men obtain relief with cognitive behavioral therapy. Some evidence also suggests that symptoms can be relieved with exercise and light physical activity. (For references, see "Prostatitis and pain syndromes," below right.)

Men might worry that prostatitis is contagious. They shouldn't. It's not contagious and can't be sexually transmitted.

Some evidence suggests that repeat biopsies for prostate cancer can increase the risk for prostatitis. But whether the longstanding inflammation associated with prostatitis increases the risk of prostate cancer over time remains uncertain. Various lines of evidence have suggested that chronic inflammation could give rise to cancer, but there is no proof of a direct connection between prostatitis and prostate cancer. (For references, see "Prostatitis and prostate cancer," page 16.) One thing to keep in mind is that prostatitis itself can increase prostate-specific antigen (PSA) levels, so men should not be alarmed if their PSA spikes during a bout of prostatitis. This doesn't necessarily signify cancer. Note that the PSA level can take months to return to its normal level (see "Prostatitis and PSA," below).

Prostatitis and PSA

When a man has either the acute or chronic bacterial form of prostatitis, prostate-specific antigen (PSA) may leak from prostate cells into the bloodstream, and a PSA test will show a large increase. A jump in PSA levels can be alarming. But if a man has prostatitis, that condition—not prostate cancer—may very well be the reason for the rise in PSA.

If an increase in PSA is caused by an infection, PSA levels will fall after the infection has cleared, although that may take three to six months. Because the PSA levels will be high, you might hold off on prostate cancer screening or having a repeat test until after you're done taking antibiotics.

If you are at high risk for prostate cancer and your PSA seems particularly high even after accounting for the possible effect of prostatitis, your doctor might recommend repeat PSA testing or a biopsy.

Diet and prostatitis

Chen X, Hu C, Peng Y, et al. Association of Diet and Lifestyle with Chronic Prostatitis/Chronic Pelvic Pain Syndrome and Pain Severity: A Case-Control Study. *Prostate Cancer and Prostatic Diseases* 2016;19(1):92–99. PMID: 26666410.

Psychological stress and prostatitis

Lien CS, Chung CJ, Lin CL, et al. Increased Risk of Prostatitis in Male Patients with Depression. *World Journal of Biological Psychiatry* 2020;21(2):111–18. PMID: 31198079.

Naliboff BD, Stephens AJ, Lai HH, et al. Clinical and Psychosocial Predictors of Urological Chronic Pelvic Pain Symptom Change in 1 Year: A Prospective Study from the MAPP Research Network. *Journal of Urology* 2017;198(4):848–57. PMID: 28528930.

Riegel B, Bruenahl CA, Ahyai S, et al. Assessing Psychological Factors, Social Aspects and Psychiatric Co-Morbidity Associated with Chronic Prostatitis/Chronic Pelvic Pain Syndrome (CP/CPPS) in Men—A Systematic Review. *Journal of Psychosomatic Research* 2014;77(5):333–50. PMID: 25300538.

Prostatitis and pain syndromes

Anderson RU, Wise D, Nathanson BH. Chronic Prostatitis and/or Chronic Pelvic Pain as a Psychoneuromuscular Disorder—A Meta-Analysis. *Urology* 2018;120:23–29. PMID: 30056195.

Gasperi M, Krieger JN, Forsberg C, et al. Chronic Prostatitis and Comorbid Non-Urological Overlapping Pain Conditions: A Co-Twin Control Study. *Journal of Psychosomatic Research* 2017;102:29–33. PMID: 28992894.

Zhang R, Chomistek AK, Dimitrakoff JD, et al. Physical Activity and Chronic Prostatitis/Chronic Pelvic Pain Syndrome. *Medicine & Science in Sports & Exercise* 2015;47(4):757–64. PMID: 25116086.

PubMed See page 120.

Diagnosing prostatitis

No single test or diagnostic procedure can confirm a case of prostatitis. If you experience urinary discomfort, such as painful or burning urination or pain in the pelvic area, your doctor will start to look for signs of inflammation and infection by performing a digital rectal exam. An inflamed prostate often feels swollen and mushy to the doctor, like an overripe piece of fruit. Pelvic imaging—performed with CT, ultrasound, or MRI—can in some cases provide additional information to help diagnose your condition. (For references, see "Imaging tests for prostatitis," below left.)

Your doctor will also have your urine tested to check for bacteria and white blood cells. If both bacteria and white blood cells are present, a bacterial infection is probably the cause, and your doctor will likely prescribe antibiotics. More often, though, only white blood cells are discovered—a sign of inflammation but not necessarily a bacterial infection. In that case, the prostatitis is classified as one of the nonbacterial types, which are more difficult to treat.

Treating prostatitis

Prostatitis is generally divided into four categories: Category I, acute bacterial prostatitis; Category II, chronic bacterial prostatitis; Category III, chronic nonbacterial prostatitis/chronic pelvic pain syndrome—which is divided into inflammatory (IIIA) and noninflammatory (IIIB) subtypes; and Category IV, asymptomatic inflammatory prostatitis. (For references, see "Prostatitis overviews," page 17.)

Category I: Acute bacterial prostatitis

Acute bacterial prostatitis, which occurs when the prostate suddenly becomes inflamed, may be caused by bacteria that normally live in the colon. The organisms get on the skin near the anus, multiply there, and then find a way to travel up the urethra and infect the prostate. *Escherichia coli* is the most common culprit, but many different kinds of bacteria can cause acute bacterial prostatitis, particularly among men with compromised immune systems. Recent advances with ultrasensitive DNA technologies make it possible to identify harmful bacteria in a man's urine and prostate secretions much more accurately. These new methods help in the selection of antibiotics that can effectively treat the infection. (For reference, see "Infections and prostatitis," page 14.)

The symptoms of acute bacterial prostatitis come on swiftly and include high fever, chills, joint and muscle aches, and profound fatigue. In addition, you may have pain around the base of the penis, behind the scrotum, and in the lower back. Some men experience an uncomfortable feeling of fullness in the rectum. As the prostate becomes more swollen, you may find it difficult to urinate, and the urine stream may dwindle to a trickle. If you can't urinate at all, it's a medical emergency. The prostate may be so swollen and inflamed that it's completely blocking urine flow. Depending on the severity of symptoms, hospitalization may be necessary.

The good news is that antibiotics are a highly effective treatment for acute bacterial prostatitis. Typically, doctors prescribe oral antibiotics in the fluoroquinolone

Prostatitis and prostate cancer

Balaban M, Ozkaptan O, Sevine L, et al. Acute Prostatitis After Prostate Biopsy Under Ciprofloxacin Prophylaxis With or Without Ornidazole and Pre-Biopsy Enema: Analysis of 3,479 Prostate Biopsy Cases. *International Brazilian Journal of Urology* 2020;46(1):60–66. PMID: 31851459.

Boehm K, Valdivieso R, Meskawi M, et al. Prostatitis, Other Genitourinary Infections and Prostate Cancer: Results from a Population-Based Case-Control Study. *World Journal of Urology* 2016;34(3):425–30. PMID: 26108732.

Cai T, Santi R, Tamanini I, et al. Current Knowledge of the Potential Links Between Inflammation and Prostate Cancer. *International Journal of Molecular Sciences* 2019;20(15):3833. PMID: 31390729.

Langston M, Horn M, Khan S, et al. A Systematic Review and Meta-Analysis of Associations Between Clinical Prostatitis and Prostate Cancer: New Estimates Accounting for Detection Bias. *Cancer Epidemiology, Biomarkers & Prevention* 2019;28(10):1594–603. PMID: 31337640.

Zhang L, Wang Y, Qin Z, et al. Correlation Between Prostatitis, Benign Prostatic Hyperplasia, and Prostate Cancer: A Systematic Review and Meta-Analysis. *Journal of Cancer* 2020;11(1):177–89. PMID: 31892984.

Imaging tests for prostatitis

Clemens JQ, Mullins C, Ackerman AL, et al. Urologic Chronic Pelvic Pain Syndrome: Insights from the MAPP Research Network. *Nature Reviews Urology* 2019;16(3):187–200. PMID: 30560936.

Clemente A, Renzulli M, Reginelli, et al. Chronic Prostatitis/Pelvic Pain Syndrome: MRI Findings and Clinical Correlations. *Andrologia* 2019;51(9):e13361. PMID: 31264247.

Shakur A, Hames K, O'Shea A, et al. Prostatitis: Imaging Appearances and Diagnostic Considerations. *Clinical Radiology* 2021;76(6):416–26. PMID: 33632522.

class, which include ciprofloxacin (Cipro), levofloxacin (Levaquin), and ofloxacin (Floxin), because in most cases, the clinical benefits outweigh the risk of side effects (see Table 1, below).

Category II: Chronic bacterial prostatitis

Chronic means lasting a long time, so chronic bacterial prostatitis is exactly what the name suggests: prostatitis caused by a bacterial infection that lingers, usually for several months. It appears to be more common in older men who have BPH. Between 5% and 10% of acute bacterial prostatitis cases develop into chronic ones. But chronic bacterial prostatitis often begins as a subtle, low-grade infection that causes moderate symptoms.

Men with chronic bacterial prostatitis are usually troubled by on-again, off-again urinary symptoms, such as a sudden urge to go or frequent urination. Some men have low back pain, rectal pain, or a feeling of heaviness behind the scrotum. Others have

Prostatitis overviews

Khan FU, Ihsan AU, Khan HU, et al. Comprehensive Overview of Prostatitis. *Biomedicine & Pharmacotherapy* 2017;94:1064–76. PMID: 28813783.

Sutcliffe S, Jemielita T, Lai HH, et al. A Case-Crossover Study of Urological Chronic Pelvic Pain Syndrome Flare Triggers in the MAPP Research Network. *Journal of Urology* 2018;199(5):1245–51. PMID: 29288643.

Zhang J, Liang C, Shang X, et al. Chronic Prostatitis/Chronic Pelvic Pain Syndrome: A Disease or Symptom? Current Perspectives on Diagnosis, Treatment, and Prognosis. *American Journal of Men's Health* 2020;14(1):epub. PMID: 32005088.

PubMed See page 120.

Table 1. Medications to treat prostatitis

Medication	Side effects	Comments
Antibiotics		
cefiximine (Suprax) ceftriaxone (Rocephin) ciprofloxacin (Cipro) fosfomycin (Monurol) levofloxacin (Levaquin) ofloxacin (Floxin) trimethoprim/sulfamethoxazole (Bactrim, Septra, Sulfatrim)	Nausea, vomiting, stomach pain, indigestion, diarrhea, upset stomach, and loss of appetite are most common. Fluoroquinolone antibiotics, including ciprofloxacin, levofloxacin, and ofloxacin, can cause permanent and severe side effects affecting the muscles and central nervous system. May also increase risk of tendinitis and tears in the Achilles tendon and in other tendons. Recent evidence also links them with aortic dissection, or tears in the inner layer of the large blood vessel branching off the heart. (For references, see "Side effects of fluoroquinolones," page 18.)	Used to treat bacterial infection (such as in Category I and Category II prostatitis); may also be tried in newly diagnosed patients with Category IIIA (inflammatory) prostatitis, based on the assumption that infection is present, even if it can't be detected in urinary cultures.
Anticholinergic drugs		
oxybutynin (Ditropan) tolterodine (Detrol)	Dry mouth, blurred vision, dry eyes or nose, dry skin, upset stomach, stomach pain, and headache are most common.	Reduce urinary urgency or leakage by decreasing bladder contractions.
Alpha blockers (nonselective)		
doxazosin (Cardura) terazosin (Hytrin)	Dizziness, headache, and fatigue are most common. Nasal congestion, dry mouth, and swelling in the ankles can also occur. Low blood pressure (hypotension), although rare, may pose a danger for some people.	Relax the muscles at the neck of the bladder, easing the flow of urine; should be used carefully by people with hypertension or heart disease.
Alpha blockers (selective)		
alfuzosin (Uroxatral) silodosin (Rapaflo) tamsulosin (Flomax)	Dizziness, headache, and fatigue are most common. Nasal congestion, dry mouth, and swelling in the ankles can also occur.	Like the nonselective drugs, relax the muscles at the neck of the bladder, easing the flow of urine; however, these do not lower blood pressure.
PDE5 inhibitor		
tadalafil (Cialis)	Flushing, headaches, dizziness, nasal congestion and muscle pain are common but generally dissipate with time. Rarely, allergic reactions occur.	Relaxes smooth muscle at the bladder neck, easing the flow of urine; used to treat severe chronic prostatitis/chronic pelvic pain syndrome.

pain after ejaculation, and the semen may be tinged with blood. As with the urinary symptoms, these symptoms wax and wane, and they are sometimes so mild that men don't notice them.

For the most part, the same types of bacteria that cause acute bacterial prostatitis cause the chronic version of the disease, and the same antibiotics—oral fluoroquinolones—are prescribed (see Table 1, page 17). A four- to six-week course usually does the trick.

However, bacterial resistance against fluoroquinolones is a growing threat, and that's driving a need for alternatives. One possibility is the antibiotic fosfomycin (Monurol), which works by blocking proteins that help build up the bacterial wall and was long used to treat urinary tract infections. Sometimes described as an old and forgotten antibiotic, in recent years it has been revived as a safe and potentially useful alternative for treating multi-drug-resistant infections. The authors of a 2020 review of 10 published studies reported that fosfomycin can be effective for prostatitis when other drugs stop working, although further studies would be helpful for establishing the optimal dosing regimen and the best ways to use the drug. (For references, see "Chronic bacterial prostatitis," at left.)

Side effects of fluoroquinolones

Richards GA, Brink AJ, Feldman C. Rational Use of Fluoroquinolones. *South African Medical Journal* 2019;109(6):378–81. PMID: 31266554.

Singh S, Nautiyal A. Aortic Dissection and Aortic Aneurysms Associated with Fluoroquinolones: A Systematic Review and Meta-Analysis. *American Journal of Medicine* 2017;130(12):1449–57. PMID: 28739200.

Chronic bacterial prostatitis

Kwan ACF, Beahm NP. Fosfomycin for Bacterial Prostatitis: A Review. *International Journal of Antimicrobial Agents.* 2020;56(4):epub. PMID: 32721595.

Lee CC, Lee MT, Chen YS, et al. Risk of Aortic Dissection and Aortic Aneurysm in Patients Taking Oral Fluoroquinolone. *JAMA Internal Medicine* 2015;175(11):1839–47. PMID: 26436523.

Magri V, Boltri M, Cai T, et al. Multidisciplinary Approach to Prostatitis. *Archives of Italian Urology and Andrology* 2019;90(4):227–48. PMID: 30655633.

Perletti G, Marras E, Wagenlehner FM, et al. Antimicrobial Therapy for Chronic Bacterial Prostatitis. *Cochrane Database of Systematic Reviews* 2013;8:CD009071. PMID: 23934982.

Su ZT, Zenilman JM, Sfanos KS, et al. Management of Chronic Bacterial Prostatitis. *Current Urology Reports* 2020;21(7):29. PMID: 32488742.

Category III: Chronic nonbacterial prostatitis / chronic pelvic pain syndrome

The most common form of prostatitis is called chronic nonbacterial prostatitis / chronic pelvic pain syndrome (CP/CPPS). The symptoms are similar to those of chronic bacterial prostatitis, but there is no evidence of a bacterial infection. The trigger may be stress, an undetectable infectious agent, or physical trauma that causes inflammation or nerve damage in the genitourinary area. Over time, the nervous system may become more sensitive. Some physicians and researchers are beginning to think that the condition may affect the entire pelvic floor—all of the muscles, nerves, and tissues that support the bladder, rectum, prostate, and other pelvic organs involved with bowel, bladder, and sexual function—not just the prostate gland. In these cases, the pelvic floor muscles can tighten up and spasm. Specialized types of physical therapy can provide some relief. However, men with CP/CPPS should avoid performing Kegel exercises (see page 114), which further tighten muscles near the prostate and can make symptoms worse.

Treatments for chronic prostatitis include the following:

- antibiotics for men whose prostatitis is preceded by a urinary tract infection
- nonsteroidal anti-inflammatory pain relievers such as aspirin and ibuprofen
- anticholinergics to reduce urinary urgency
- alpha blockers to relax smooth muscles in the bladder neck and prostate, thus reducing muscle tightness and spasms that can prevent normal urine flow
- PDE5 inhibitors to improve blood flow to the prostate and relax the organ
- acupuncture to control pain pathways and promote the release of your body's own pain-relieving compounds, such as enkephalins and endorphins.

A study presented at the annual meeting of the American Urological Association in 2018 showed promising results in patients with CP/CPPS who were treated with fluoroquinolones and another drug called tadalafil (Cialis), one of a class of drugs known as PDE5 inhibitors, which are ordinarily used for treating erectile dysfunction and BPH. The researchers theorized that because tadalafil improves blood flow to pelvic organs, it would help the antibiotic penetrate into affected tissues and improve the clearance of inflammatory compounds. After four weeks of the combined treatment, patients reported greater reductions in pain, urinary symptoms, and erectile functioning than patients treated with the antibiotic alone. The study has not been published in full or undergone peer review. However, Dr. Marc Garnick, editor in chief of the *Annual*, says that his clinical experience supports the study's conclusions.

A more recent study with 25 men, published in 2020, showed some improvements with tadalafil treatment by itself. The men were treated for an average of 15 months, suggesting that long-term therapy can lead to sustained improvements in CP/CPPS symptoms.

Acupuncture has also shown long-lasting clinical benefits, according to the results of a randomized clinical trial reported in 2021. During this study, which enrolled 440 men with moderate to severe CP/CPPS, 20 acupuncture sessions over eight weeks resulted in symptom improvements that were still holding up six months after treatment. A literature review published in 2019 also supported acupuncture therapy. (For references, see "Treatment for CP/CPPS," at right.)

Category IV: Asymptomatic inflammatory prostatitis

This form of the disease has no symptoms. It is diagnosed when white blood cells are found in prostate secretions or in prostate tissue during an evaluation for other prostate disorders. Given that it creates no problems and has no known cause, doctors do not treat it.

Treatment for CP/CPPS

El Sayed AA, Dosyky H, Marouf A, et al. Daily Low Dose Tadalafil in Treatment of Chronic Prostatitis/Chronic Pelvic Pain Syndrome: Randomized Controlled Study of Efficacy and Safety. Presented at the 2018 Annual Meeting of the American Urological Association, San Francisco, CA. Abstract No. PD62-01.

Magistro G, Wagenlehner FM, Grabe M, et al. Contemporary Management of Chronic Prostatitis/Chronic Pelvic Pain Syndrome. *European Urology* 2016;69(2):286–97. PMID: 26411805.

Pineault K, Roy S, Gabrielson A, et al. Phosphodiesterase Type 5 Inhibitor Therapy Provides Sustained Relief of Symptoms in Patients with Chronic Pelvic Pain Syndrome. *Translational Urology and Andrology* 2020;9(2):391–97. PMID: 32420144.

Pirola GM, Veracchi T, Rosadi S, et al. Chronic Prostatitis: Current Treatment Options. *Research and Reports in Urology* 2019;11:165–74. PMID: 31240202.

Rees J, Abrahams M, Doble A, et al. Diagnosis and Treatment of Chronic Bacterial Prostatitis and Chronic Prostatitis/Chronic Pelvic Pain Syndrome: A Consensus Guideline. *BJU International* 2015;116(4):509–25. PMID: 25711488.

Sandhu J, Tu HYV. Recent Advances in Managing Chronic Prostatitis/Chronic Pelvic Pain Syndrome. *F1000Research* 2017;6(F1000 Faculty Rev):1747. PMID: 29034074.

Sun Y, Liu Y, Liu B, et al. Efficacy of Acupuncture for Chronic Prostatitis/Chronic Pelvic Pain Syndrome: A Randomized Trial. *Annals of Internal Medicine* 2021; 174(10):1357–66. PMID: 34399062.

Wazir J, Ullah R, Li S, et al. Efficacy of Acupuncture in the Treatment of Chronic Prostatitis–Chronic Pelvic Pain Syndrome: A Review of the Literature. *International Urology and Nephrology* 2019;51(12):2093–106. PMID: 31468287.

Zaidi N, Thomas D, Chughtai B. Management of Chronic Prostatitis (CP). *Current Urology Reports* 2018;19(11):88. PMID: 30167899.

PubMed See page 120.

4

Prostate enlargement (benign prostatic hyperplasia)

Getting this "going"—and "growing"—problem under control

Lifestyle factors and BPH

Das K, Buchholz N. Benign Prostate Hyperplasia and Nutrition. *Clinical Nutrition ESPEN* 2019;33:5–11. PMID: 31451276.

Launer BM, McVary KT, Ricke WA, et al. The Rising Worldwide Impact of Benign Prostatic Hyperplasia. *British Journal of Urology International* 2021;127(6):722–28. PMID: 33124118.

Lloyd GL, Marks JM, Ricke WA. Benign Prostatic Hyperplasia and Lower Urinary Tract Symptoms: What is the Role and Significance of Inflammation? *Current Urology Reports* 2019;20(9):54. PMID: 31377881.

Silva V, Grande AJ, Peccin MS. Physical Activity for Lower Urinary Tract Symptoms Secondary to Benign Prostatic Obstruction. *Cochrane Database of Systematic Reviews* 2019;4:CD012044. PMID: 30953341.

Wolin KY, Grubb RL 3rd, Pakpahan R, et al. Physical Activity and Benign Prostatic Hyperplasia-Related Outcomes and Nocturia. *Medicine & Science in Sports & Exercise* 2015;47(3):581–92. PMID: 25010403.

PubMed See page 120.

The normal prostate in men ages 20 to 30 weighs approximately 20 grams—less than an ounce. But from around the time of a man's 50th birthday (sometimes earlier), his prostate begins to grow, often reaching 50 to 100 grams by the time he turns 80. In some men, it grows even more. Weights of over 500 grams have been recorded.

This natural enlargement is called benign prostatic hyperplasia (BPH). It is called benign because it is not cancerous, and hyperplasia is the medical term for an increase in the number of cells in a tissue or an organ. If a man lives long enough, he will almost certainly experience some degree of BPH. Indeed, as the global population ages, BPH imposes an increasing human burden that far exceeds that of other urological diseases. Although it does not lead to prostate cancer, the two problems can coexist.

Between 50% and 60% of men with BPH never develop symptoms, while others find that BPH can make life miserable, causing lower urinary tract symptoms, or LUTS (see "Lots of LUTS: Symptoms of BPH," page 21), that lead them to seek treatment. That said, BPH is not considered to be a health problem unless it results in LUTS or other mechanical problems, such as the development of bladder stones or ruptured blood vessels.

Apart from age, risk factors for BPH include abdominal obesity, diabetes, high blood pressure (hypertension), inflammation of the prostate (prostatitis), and a lack of physical activity. Diet also seems to matter. Several large studies have found a correlation between Western dietary patterns (high intake of red meat, refined grains, and sugar) and prostate enlargement. (For references, see "Lifestyle factors and BPH," at left.)

How BPH progresses

As the prostate enlarges, it starts to press against the urethra and the bladder, like a foot stepping on a garden hose or fingers pinching a straw (see Figure 2, page 21). This pressure eventually obstructs the flow of urine, forcing the bladder to squeeze harder to push urine through the urethra. But straining to urinate, although unavoidable, only makes matters worse. Like any muscle, the bladder wall becomes thicker with work. That thickness reduces the amount of urine the bladder can hold and causes it to contract even when it contains only small amounts of urine, causing more frequent urination.

The narrowing of the urethra and resultant difficulty in emptying the bladder cause many of the problems associated with BPH. You may feel as though you have to urinate immediately, yet you strain to do so. You may have a weak urinary stream or one that stops and starts. You may dribble after urinating or feel as if you're not emptying your bladder completely. And you may feel the need to urinate frequently—even every few minutes; at night, the continual need to go to the bathroom can make it impossible to sleep well, causing all sorts of adverse health consequences. Some men also experience urinary incontinence, the involuntary discharge of urine.

Most physicians advise against medical or surgical treatment for men with mild symptoms because the side effects of the treatment outweigh the potential benefits. But if the symptoms worsen, ordinary activities may become a challenge. A man may find it hard to sit through a lengthy meeting. Aisle seats become a necessity so there's a quick escape to the bathroom. Many men wear absorbent pads or limit themselves to dark clothing to conceal their incontinence.

BPH can also result in some serious complications. If an enlarged prostate keeps your bladder from emptying completely, you may be vulnerable to frequent urinary tract infections. The risk of developing bladder stones increases. A growing prostate can rupture blood vessels in the urethra, causing blood to appear in the urine. A thorough medical evaluation is necessary any time there's blood in the urine.

If obstructive BPH goes untreated for too long, muscles in the bladder wall may weaken. Your bladder may not have enough power to push urine past the obstructing prostate gland, a condition known as acute urinary retention. The bladder may become so stretched out that urine cannot adequately empty from the kidneys. In the worst cases, this can lead to kidney failure.

Lots of LUTS: Symptoms of BPH

The most common symptoms of BPH involve changes or problems with urination. In medical articles, they are often grouped together and referred to as LUTS, which stands for lower urinary tract symptoms. They include

- a hesitant, interrupted, or weak urine stream
- urgency, leaking, or dribbling
- a sense of incomplete emptying
- more frequent urination, especially at night.

Note that while many men with BPH have LUTS, there are other causes of LUTS, so not all men with LUTS have BPH.

Figure 2. An inside look at BPH

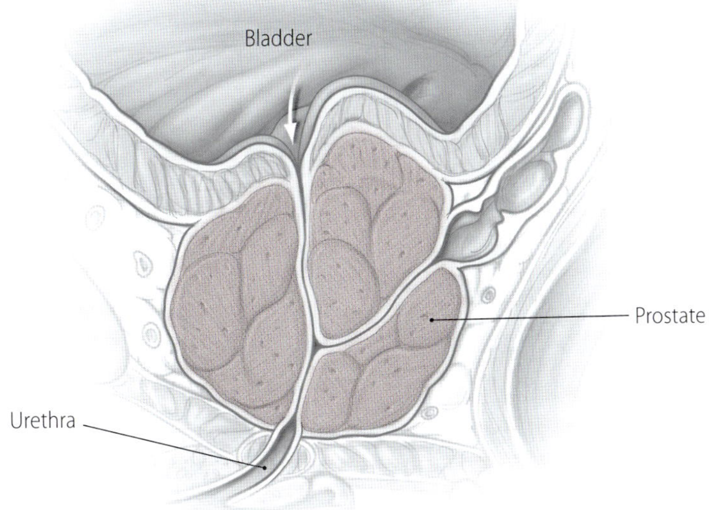

As the prostate gland enlarges, it constricts the urethra, the tube that carries urine out of the body, and impedes urine flow. The bladder has to work harder to force stored urine out (see arrow). Over time, the bladder walls thicken, leaving less room for urine.

Not being able to urinate at all is painful and a true medical emergency, requiring the temporary passage of a catheter (a thin tube) through the urethra to allow the bladder to drain. Fortunately, such complications are uncommon because most men seek medical attention well before serious problems develop.

Diagnosing BPH

If you experience the symptoms of BPH, see your doctor. Be aware that BPH symptoms can overlap with those of other conditions, such as an overactive bladder, as well as prostate cancer. Expect questions about your urinary flow problems, how long the symptoms have been present, and any prior genitourinary surgery or procedures. You will probably be asked about your health habits and the medications you are taking. For instance, drugs that have antihistamine effects can cause urinary symptoms because they affect the muscle in the wall of the bladder.

Your doctor may also ask you to complete a questionnaire, such as the International Prostate Symptom Score, to help evaluate the severity of your BPH (see "Your urinary symptom score," page 23).

An adequate physical exam and diagnostic workup includes a post-void residual urine test (which measures the amount of urine left in the bladder after you use the bathroom), a digital rectal examination (DRE; see page 44) and, if you and your doctor agree, a prostate-specific antigen (PSA) test (see page 44). It also includes several other laboratory tests, such as urinalysis, which allows your doctor to rule out bacterial infections and look for untreated diabetes (another possible cause of frequent urination, particularly at night).

Treating BPH

Often a man's lifestyle will determine how burdensome he finds BPH. The symptoms that disrupt the daily activities of a man who is conducting business or traveling may not bother another man who spends much of his day at home within easy reach of a bathroom. When symptoms are not particularly bothersome, you and your doctor may elect to hold off on treatment and instead monitor your BPH. To determine if this is the right choice for you, your doctor may ask if your symptoms prevent you from engaging in enjoyable activities, if they appear to be worsening, or if you are ready to accept a small degree of risk in exchange for the benefits of treatment.

For more troubling symptoms, most doctors begin by recommending a combination of lifestyle changes (see "Tips for relieving BPH symptoms," page 24) and medication (see Table 2, page 25). Often these approaches will be enough to relieve the worst symptoms, so you won't need surgery.

Should surgery become necessary, keep in mind that there are several surgical procedures available, including newer, noninvasive techniques that are generally well tolerated. Before proceeding, check with your health insurance company to make sure your choice is covered.

continued on page 24

Your urinary symptom score

To evaluate the severity of your benign prostatic hyperplasia (BPH), your doctor may ask you to complete a questionnaire like the International Prostate Symptom Score (IPSS). Choose one number to respond to questions 1 to 7, and then calculate your total urinary symptom score. Question 8 is separate and indicates how bothered you are by the condition.

Urinary symptom scores of 1–7 indicate mild symptoms. Scores of 8–18 are considered moderate. And scores of 19 or greater are severe. If you have moderate to severe symptoms, and if your answer to question 8 is a 3, 4, or 5, you may want to discuss treatment (either medication or surgery) with your physician.

1. Over the past month, how often have you had a sensation of not having emptied your bladder completely after you finished urinating?

- 0 ○ Not at all
- 1 ○ Less than 1 in 5 times
- 2 ○ Less than half the time
- 3 ○ About half the time
- 4 ○ More than half the time
- 5 ○ Almost always

2. Over the past month, how often have you had to urinate again less than two hours after you last finished urinating?

- 0 ○ Not at all
- 1 ○ Less than 1 in 5 times
- 2 ○ Less than half the time
- 3 ○ About half the time
- 4 ○ More than half the time
- 5 ○ Almost always

3. Over the past month, how often have you stopped and started again several times while urinating?

- 0 ○ Not at all
- 1 ○ Less than 1 in 5 times
- 2 ○ Less than half the time
- 3 ○ About half the time
- 4 ○ More than half the time
- 5 ○ Almost always

4. Over the past month, how often have you found it difficult to postpone urination?

- 0 ○ Not at all
- 1 ○ Less than 1 in 5 times
- 2 ○ Less than half the time
- 3 ○ About half the time
- 4 ○ More than half the time
- 5 ○ Almost always

5. Over the past month, how often have you had a weak urinary stream?

- 0 ○ Not at all
- 1 ○ Less than 1 in 5 times
- 2 ○ Less than half the time
- 3 ○ About half the time
- 4 ○ More than half the time
- 5 ○ Almost always

6. Over the past month, how often have you had to push or strain to begin urination?

- 0 ○ Not at all
- 1 ○ Less than 1 in 5 times
- 2 ○ Less than half the time
- 3 ○ About half the time
- 4 ○ More than half the time
- 5 ○ Almost always

7. Over the past month, how many times, typically, did you get up to urinate between the time you went to bed and the time you got up in the morning?

- 0 ○ None
- 1 ○ Once
- 2 ○ Twice
- 3 ○ Three times
- 4 ○ Four times
- 5 ○ Five times or more

Urinary symptom score: ______

8. How would you feel if you had to live with your urinary condition the way it is now, no better, no worse, for the rest of your life?

- 0 ○ Delighted
- 1 ○ Pleased
- 2 ○ Mostly satisfied
- 3 ○ Mixed
- 4 ○ Mostly not satisfied
- 5 ○ Unhappy

Quality of life score: ______

continued from page 22

Medications approved specifically to treat BPH

Before suggesting surgery, your doctor is likely to recommend medication for BPH (see Table 2, page 25). The FDA has approved three types of drugs for BPH:

- alpha blockers, including alfuzosin (Uroxatral), doxazosin (Cardura), prazosin (Minipress), silodosin (Rapaflo), tamsulosin (Flomax), and terazosin (Hytrin)
- 5-alpha-reductase inhibitors, including dutasteride (Avodart) and finasteride (Proscar)
- the phosphodiesterase-5 (PDE5) inhibitor tadalafil (Cialis).

The FDA has also approved Jalyn, a combination of the 5-alpha-reductase inhibitor dutasteride and an alpha blocker, tamsulosin. These drugs work in different ways to alleviate urinary symptoms, and they often work well together.

A good way to think about the difference between alpha blockers and 5-alpha-reductase inhibitors is that alpha blockers target the "going" problem while 5-alpha-reductase inhibitors target the "growing" problem. Alpha blockers help with the act of urination (the "going" problem) by relaxing certain muscles in the prostate and bladder. The 5-alpha-reductase inhibitors reduce the encroachment of the prostate on the urethra and the lower part of the bladder (the "growing" problem) by decreasing the size of the prostate.

PDE5 inhibitors are a class of drugs normally used to treat erectile dysfunction, but they also help to relax muscles in the bladder neck (which connects the bladder to the urethra), and some men who take these medications also find that their urinary symptoms improve. The PDE5 inhibitor tadalafil is approved for both erectile dysfunction and BPH. When used to treat BPH (with or without erectile dysfunction), the medication is taken at a 2.5- or 5-milligram (mg) dose once daily. (Doses used solely for treating erectile dysfunction can range up to 20 mg per use.)

continued on page 26

Tips for relieving BPH symptoms

These simple steps can help alleviate some of the symptoms of BPH:

- Reduce stress by exercising regularly and practicing relaxation techniques such as meditation. Some men who are nervous and tense urinate more frequently.
- When you go to the bathroom, take the time to empty as much of your bladder as you can. This will reduce the need for subsequent trips to the toilet and minimize the chances that urine will collect and become stagnant in the bladder, leading to possible infections and bladder stones.
- Talk with your doctor about all your prescription and over-the-counter medications; some, such as antihistamines and decongestants, may affect urination. Your doctor may be able to adjust dosages, change your schedule for taking these drugs, or prescribe different medications that cause fewer urinary problems.
- Avoid drinking fluids in the evening, particularly caffeinated and alcoholic beverages. Both can affect the muscle tone of the bladder and stimulate the kidneys to produce urine, leading to nighttime urination.
- On long airplane flights, avoid drinking alcohol, and try to urinate every 60 to 90 minutes.

Table 2. Medications for BPH

Medication	Side effects	Comments
Alpha blockers (nonselective)		
doxazosin (Cardura) terazosin (Hytrin)	Dizziness, headache, and fatigue are most common. Nasal congestion, dry mouth, and swelling in the ankles can also occur. Low blood pressure (hypotension), although rare, may pose a danger for some people.	Should be used carefully by those with high blood pressure (hypertension) or heart disease. May increase risk of aggressive prostate cancer; important to monitor PSA (see "5-alpha-reductase inhibitors, alpha blockers, and cancer," page 28).
Alpha blockers (selective)		
alfuzosin (Uroxatral) prazosin (Minipress) silodosin (Rapaflo) tamsulosin (Flomax)	Dizziness, headache, and fatigue are most common. Nasal congestion, dry mouth, and swelling in the ankles can also occur. Can cause rash.	Do not lower blood pressure, but men taking silodosin may notice a drop in blood pressure upon standing.
5-alpha-reductase inhibitors		
dutasteride (Avodart) finasteride (Proscar)	Although uncommon, decreased libido, decreased ejaculate volume, and impotence may occur. (Problems with libido may continue after you stop taking finasteride.) Cardiovascular effects and depression may occur in some men. Minor reports of rash. New data suggest a heightened risk of osteoporosis.	Help shrink larger prostate glands. Reduce need for surgery. Not beneficial for small prostates. Slow to act; can take up to two years to see full benefits. Can lower PSA levels by 50%. May increase risk of aggressive prostate cancer; important to monitor PSA (see "5-alpha-reductase inhibitors, alpha blockers, and cancer," page 28). In some men, finasteride can lead to problems in sexual function, depression, and other changes in mood.
Combination therapy		
dutasteride and tamsulosin (Jalyn)	Dizziness, headache, and fatigue are most common. Low blood pressure, although rare, may pose a danger for some.	Can lower PSA levels considerably. May increase risk of aggressive prostate cancer; important to monitor PSA.
PDE5 inhibitor		
tadalafil (Cialis)	Headache, flushing, upset stomach, and nasal congestion can occur. Temporary disturbances in color vision are possible. In rare cases, may cause priapism, an erection that lasts too long.	Do not take more than one pill in 24 hours. Do not take if you are also taking alpha blockers or nitrate medications, to avoid risk of low blood pressure that can cause fainting.
Antimuscarinics		
fesoterodine (Toviaz) oxybutynin (Ditropan) tolderodine (Detrol)	Dry mouth, dilation of pupils and sensitivity to light, increased fluid pressure in the eye, and dry skin may occur.	May accelerate existing cognitive decline in the elderly.
Antidiuretic hormone		
desmopressin acetate (Noctiva)	Dizziness is the most problematic, potentially leading to falls. Others include nasal discomfort, cold symptoms, increased blood pressure, and back pain.	Nasal spray to limit nighttime urination. Can depress sodium levels in blood. Should not be taken by men with low sodium levels, as excessively low values can lead to dizziness, fainting, and coma in rare instances. Should not be taken by men with heart failure or uncontrolled hypertension.

continued from page 24

Evidence to date shows that alpha blockers, 5-alpha-reductase inhibitors, and PDE5 inhibitors are all generally safe and well tolerated for BPH treatment. (For references, see "Medications for BPH: Overviews," at left.)

Following is a more detailed discussion of each type of BPH drug.

Alpha blockers. For men with moderate enlargement of the prostate and moderate urinary problems that are too bothersome not to treat, doctors often first prescribe an alpha blocker. Alpha blocker is shorthand for alpha adrenergic–receptor antagonist, a type of medication that was originally approved to treat high blood pressure. Alpha blockers relax smooth muscle tissue by blocking the receptors that receive chemical signals instructing the tissue to contract. In the prostate, this relaxation of smooth muscle means that the prostate's "grip" on the urethra loosens, allowing urine to flow more freely.

Alpha blockers come in two forms: selective and nonselective. Because the nonselective alpha blockers—doxazosin and terazosin—can lower blood pressure, they may not be the best choice for men who are already taking a blood pressure medication. Taking several blood pressure medications at once can cause an excessive drop in blood pressure that makes people faint or get dizzy, especially when getting up from a chair or out of bed (orthostatic hypotension). Sudden episodes of low blood pressure can be dangerous for men with vascular disease, placing them at high risk for a heart attack or stroke. By contrast, the selective alpha blockers (alfuzosin, prazosin, silodosin, and tamsulosin) concentrate in the prostate, so they don't lower blood pressure, making them useful for men for whom blood pressure reduction causes problems. A 2021 review of articles published during the preceding decade concluded that alfuzosin, for instance, is effective and safe for men who are also taking drugs for high blood pressure, and that the drug also has fewer sexual side effects than nonselective alpha blockers.

Other side effects of alpha blockers include ankle swelling, nasal stuffiness, and retrograde ejaculation, when semen flows back into the bladder rather than out through the urethra. (Although it is considered a sexual side effect of BPH treatment, retrograde ejaculation does not affect the pleasurable sensations of orgasm.) Ejaculate volume is another issue with some alpha blockers. One study found that tamsulosin decreased ejaculate volume in almost 90% of men.

Alpha blockers are all reasonably effective. A 2019 review article concluded that among the alpha blockers, silodosin was most effective at reducing LUTS and improving urinary flow rates. However, the drug frequently caused problems with ejaculation, especially among men who reported the greatest benefits. And a 2018 study found that while improvements in urinary symptoms from silodosin treatment were still holding up after two years, the drug's effectiveness was also wearing off, especially in men with prostates weighing 40 grams or more. (For references, see "Alpha blockers for BPH," at left.)

Side effects from alpha blockers vary more from man to man than they do from drug to drug, so there can be a fair amount of trial and error before an individual patient finds the right one. Also, health plans may limit choices or make some medica-

Medications for BPH: Overviews

Abreu-Mendes P, Silva J, Cruz F. Pharmacology of the Lower Urinary Tract: Update on LUTS Treatment. *Therapeutic Advances in Urology* 2020;12:epub. PMID: 32489425.

Yu Z, Yan H, Xu F, et al. Efficacy and Side Effects of Drugs Commonly Used for the Treatment of Lower Urinary Symptoms Associated with Benign Prostatic Hyperplasia. *Frontiers in Pharmacology* 2020;11:658. PMID: 32457631.

Yuan JQ, Mao C, Wong SY, et al. Comparative Effectiveness and Safety of Monodrug Therapies for Lower Urinary Tract Symptoms Associated with Benign Prostatic Hyperplasia: A Network Meta-Analysis. *Medicine (Baltimore)* 2015;94(27):e974. PMID: 26166130.

Alpha blockers for BPH

DeLay KJ, Nutt M, McVary KT. Ejaculatory Dysfunction in the Treatment of Lower Urinary Tract Symptoms. *Translational Andrology and Urology* 2016;5(4):450–59. PMID: 27652217.

MacDonald R, Brasure M, Dahm P, et al. Efficacy of Newer Medications for Lower Urinary Tract Symptoms Attributed to Benign Prostatic Hyperplasia: A Systematic Review. *Aging Male* 2019;22(1):1–11. PMID: 29394114.

Mari A, Antonelli A, Cindolo L, et al. Alfuzosin for the Medical Treatment of Benign Prostatic Hyperplasia and Lower Urinary Tract Symptoms: A Systematic Review of the Literature and Narrative Synthesis. *Therapeutic Advances in Urology* 2021;13:epub. PMID: 33912246.

Matsukawa Y, Takai S, Majima T, et al. Two-year Follow up of Silodosin on Lower Urinary Tract Functions and Symptoms in Patients with Benign Prostatic Hyperplasia Based on Prostate Size: A Prospective Investigation Using Urodynamics. *Therapeutic Advances in Urology* 2018;10(9):263–72. PMID: 30116302.

tions more expensive than others. All of this means that working with your doctor can be a key component of successful treatment.

5-alpha-reductase inhibitors. The two FDA-approved 5-alpha-reductase inhibitors, dutasteride and finasteride, shrink the prostate, but they are relatively slow in having an effect and do not relieve urinary symptoms as readily as the alpha blockers. Drugs in this class can also be used to prevent LUTS in asymptomatic men with enlarged prostates.

5-alpha-reductase inhibitors work by altering hormone ratios within the prostate. Specifically, they interfere with the action of 5-alpha reductase, an enzyme that converts the well-known male hormone testosterone to its lesser-known relative, dihydrotestosterone (DHT). As a result of that interference, DHT levels in the prostate decline. Because DHT is an important player in the processes involved in prostate growth, the gland slowly shrinks, leading to improvements in urinary symptoms within two to three months. The same hormonal effects also make 5-alpha-reductase inhibitors useful for treating hair loss.

A review of six studies, published in 2020, found that dutasteride was associated with better patient-reported symptom scores. Yet finasteride and dutasteride were also shown to reduce prostate size comparably and improve urine flow and retention rates similarly, with no difference in side effects.

In men who don't have prostate cancer, dutasteride and finasteride tend to lower PSA levels by about 50%. For that reason, it's important to obtain a baseline PSA value before you begin treatment with a 5-alpha-reductase inhibitor and then measure the level again after six months to a year to see the difference. If the PSA level hasn't decreased by about the expected 50%, or if it rises, you may need a biopsy to determine if this is a sign of cancer. Conversely, if you're screened for prostate cancer while taking a 5-alpha-reductase inhibitor—and you haven't obtained a baseline value—then the measured PSA level should be doubled to correct for the drug's PSA-lowering effects. Otherwise, the reading will be deceptively low. Indeed, a 2019 study found higher rates of advanced cancer in men taking 5-alpha-reductase inhibitors for BPH, which the authors attributed to delayed diagnoses arising from artificially low PSA screening results.

Treatment with finasteride and dutasteride, especially in elderly patients, can also have troubling side effects, including depressed mood. In 2021, researchers citing data on adverse drug reactions collected by the World Health Organization reported that finasteride, in particular, was associated with higher risks of suicidal thinking and various other psychological problems in men younger than 45 who had used the drug as a hair loss treatment. Other symptoms associated with 5-alpha-reductase inhibitors include erectile dysfunction, fatigue, and sleep disturbances. Sexual side effects can persist, sometimes for months, after men stop taking the drugs. In studies, these affect only a small minority of men—less than 10%. But doctors say that in actual practice, sexual side effects are much more common, affecting up to a third of their patients.

That said, it's possible to mitigate the erectile side effects of 5-alpha-reductase inhibitors by adding the PDE5 inhibitor tadalafil. A 2015 review of the medical literature concluded that finasteride and tadalafil are suitable in combination, especially for

5-alpha-reductase inhibitors for BPH

Basaria S, Jasuja R, Huang G, et al. Characteristics of Men Who Report Persistent Sexual Symptoms After Finasteride Use for Hair Loss. *Journal of Clinical Endocrinology & Metabolism* 2016;101(12):4669–80. PMID: 27662439.

Bortnick E, Brown C, Simma-Chiang V, et al. Modern Best Practice in the Management of Benign Prostatic Hyperplasia in the Elderly. *Therapeutic Advances in Urology* 2020;12:epub. PMID: 32547642.

Diviccaro S, Giatti S, Borgo F, et al. Treatment of Male Rats with Finasteride, an Inhibitor of 5Alpha-Reductase Enzyme, Induces Long-Lasting Effects on Depressive-Like Behavior, Hippocampal Neurogenesis, Neuroinflammation and Gut Microbiota Composition. *Psychoneuroendocrinology* 2019;99:206–15. PMID: 30265917.

Elkelany OO, Owen RC, Kim ED. Combination of Tadalafil and Finasteride for Improving the Symptoms of Benign Prostatic Hyperplasia: Critical Appraisal and Patient Focus. *Therapeutics and Clinical Risk Management* 2015;11:507–13. PMID: 25848297.

Kim JH, Shim SR, Khandwala Y, et al. Risk of Depression After 5 Alpha Reductase Inhibitor Medication: Meta-Analysis. *World Journal of Men's Health* 2020;38(4):535–44. PMID: 31190484.

Nguyen DD, Marchese M, Cone EB, et al. Investigation of Suicidality and Psychological Adverse Events in Patients Treated with Finasteride. *JAMA Dermatology* 2021;157(1):35–42. PMID: 33175100.

Sarkar RR, Parsons JK, Bryant AK, et al. Association of Treatment with 5α-Reductase Inhibitors with Time to Diagnosis and Mortality in Prostate Cancer. *JAMA Internal Medicine* 2019;179(6):812–19. PMID: 31058923.

Wallner LP, DiBello JR, Li BH, et al. The Use of 5-Alpha Reductase Inhibitors to Manage Benign Prostatic Hyperplasia and the Risk of All-Cause Mortality. *Urology* 2018;119:70–78. PMID: 29906480.

Zhou Z, Cui Y, Wu J, et al. Efficacy and Safety of Dutasteride Compared with Finasteride in Treating Males with Benign Prostatic Hyperplasia: A Meta-Analysis of Randomized Controlled Trials. *Experimental Therapeutic Medicine* 2020;20(2):1566–74. PMID: 32742388.

PubMed See page 120.

men with moderate to severe BPH. (For references, see "5-alpha-reductase inhibitors for BPH," page 27.)

Combination therapy. Because alpha blockers and 5-alpha-reductase inhibitors work differently, they often control urinary symptoms more effectively when taken together rather than by themselves. That's especially true for men with very large prostates. When a doxazosin-finasteride combination was tested in a large trial, it was more effective than either medication alone at preventing LUTS from getting worse. However, a 2016 analysis of five published studies enrolling over 6,000 men in total found the combination was also more likely to cause sexual side effects. It was a similar story with tamsulosin-dutasteride, sold as Jalyn. (For references, see "Combination therapy for BPH," at left.)

PDE5 inhibitors. Studies have established a physiological link between erectile dysfunction and the urinary symptoms that accompany BPH. Prescribed for erectile dysfunction, PDE5 inhibitors—including sildenafil (Viagra) and vardenafil (Levitra), as well as tadalafil (Cialis)—relax smooth muscle in the bladder neck, urethra, and prostate, and they also improve erectile function, urinary symptoms, and quality of life in men with both conditions.

Tadalafil is approved by the FDA as a stand-alone treatment for BPH-related urinary symptoms and as a dual treatment to address both BPH and erectile dysfunction. A study published in 2020 showed that daily treatment with tadalafil was as effective as tamsulosin in treating moderate to severe BPH symptoms, and another 2020 study showed the drug lessened the frequency of having to get up to urinate at night. Combining the two drugs is also an option: in 2019, physicians reported that tadalafil given along with the alpha blocker tamsulosin relieved urinary symptoms more effectively than tadalafil by itself, and a 2020 review article found that it did so without compromising sexual functioning. Still, tadalafil can reduce blood flow to the heart, so experts

Combination therapy for BPH

Favilla V, Russo GI, Privitera S, et al. Impact of Combination Therapy 5-Alpha Reductase Inhibitors (5-ARI) Plus Alpha-Blockers (AB) on Erectile Dysfunction and Decrease of Libido in Patients with LUTS/BPH: A Systematic Review with Meta-Analysis. *Aging Male* 2016;19(3):175–81. PMID: 27310433.

Zitoun OA, Farhat AM, Mohamed MA, et al. Management of Benign Prostate Hyperplasia (BPH) by Combinatorial Approach Using Alpha-1-Adrenergic Antagonists and 5-Alpha-Reductase Inhibitors. *European Journal of Pharmacology* 2020;883:epub. PMID: 32592768.

Tadalafil for BPH

Brock GB, McVary KT, Roehrborn CG, et al. Direct Effects of Tadalafil on Lower Urinary Tract Symptoms Versus Indirect Effects Mediated Through Erectile Dysfunction Symptom Improvement: Integrated Data Analyses from 4 Placebo Controlled Clinical Studies. *Journal of Urology* 2014;191(2):405–11. PMID: 24096120.

Chapple CR, Roehrborn CG, McVary K, et al. Effect of Tadalafil on Male Lower Urinary Tract Symptoms: An Integrated Analysis of Storage and Voiding International Prostate Symptom Subscores from Four Randomised Controlled Trials. *European Urology* 2015:67(1):114–22. PMID: 25301757.

continued on page 29

5-alpha-reductase inhibitors, alpha blockers, and cancer

In addition to treating BPH, 5-alpha-reductase inhibitors have also been tested as a means of preventing prostate cancer. In two separate trials, finasteride and dutasteride were shown to lower the overall risk of prostate cancer by about 25% to 30%. Here's the catch (and it is an important one): both medications were also associated with a small, but statistically significant, increase in risks for high-grade prostate cancer. As a result, the FDA put a cancer warning on the drugs. In 2019, scientists followed up with findings showing that alpha blockers similarly reduce the likelihood of developing prostate cancer—in this case, by 11%. But increased risks of high-grade prostate cancer among diagnosed men were also observed.

If you are taking a 5-alpha-reductase inhibitor, an alpha blocker, or the combination pill Jalyn (which contains dutasteride along with the alpha blocker tamsulosin) for BPH, talk with your doctor about the cancer risk and what you should do.

Sources: Thompson IM Jr, Goodman PJ, Tangen CM, et al. Long-Term Survival of Participants in the Prostate Cancer Prevention Trial. *New England Journal of Medicine* 2013;369(7):603–10. PMID: 23944298.

Van Rompay MI, Nickel JC, Ranganathan G, et al. Impact of 5α-Reductase Inhibitor and α-Blocker Therapy for Benign Prostatic Hyperplasia on Prostate Cancer Incidence and Mortality. *BJU International* 2019;123(3):511–18. PMID: 30216624.

Walsh PC. Survival in the Prostate Cancer Prevention Trial. *New England Journal of Medicine* 2013;369(20):1967–68. PMID: 24224633.

advise against prescribing the drug to men with heart problems. (For references, see "Tadalafil for BPH," starting on page 28.)

Antimuscarinics

Some men with BPH also have overactive bladders. Symptoms include frequent urination (over eight times a day) and strong urges to urinate right away. Drugs called antimuscarinics block receptors in the smooth muscle tissue in the wall of the bladder so that this muscle is less likely to contract. Antimuscarinics include oxybutynin (Ditropan), tolterodine (Detrol), and fesoterodine (Toviaz). A 2017 study showed that men are more likely to stick with alpha blocker treatment if they're also combining it with an antimuscarinic. Experts advise caution when prescribing antimuscarinics in the elderly since the drugs can accelerate existing cognitive decline. Antimuscarinics are not approved by the FDA for use in BPH treatment. (For references, see "Antimuscarinics for overactive bladder in men with BPH," below right.)

Antidiuretic hormone

In 2017, the FDA approved a nasal spray called desmopressin acetate (Noctiva) as treatment for adults who wake up at least twice per night to urinate. This distressing problem, called nocturia, can be caused by a variety of medical conditions, such as diabetes, overactive bladder, and BPH. Desmopressin is a synthetic version of a hormone, vasopressin, which retains fluid in the body and decreases your need to urinate. The drug must be used with caution and patients should be checked regularly for low blood sodium, a possible effect of the drug that can cause confusion and a tendency to fall.

Herbal remedies

Dr. Marc Garnick, editor in chief of the *Annual*, says that there is little reason to believe that any herbal remedies (including saw palmetto and beta sitosterol) are effective, since none of the randomized trials to date have shown any benefit. They are probably not worth the money, and therefore they are not covered here.

Surgical options and tissue ablation

If the results of lifestyle changes and medication or other therapies are not satisfactory, you and your doctor will need to determine whether surgery or another procedure may be right for you. In the past, if BPH symptoms were severe—or if they were modest but still disrupted a patient's life—doctors almost universally recommended a surgical procedure called transurethral resection of the prostate (TURP). Although TURP (rhymes with burp) is still widely used and is considered the standard that alternatives should be judged against, there are plenty of other less invasive options these days that may have some advantages over TURP. Like TURP, most of them involve removing prostate tissue to reduce pressure on the urethra. The variation is in the technology used to remove that tissue.

Explanations of the most common procedures follow. (For a comparison of procedures, see Table 3, page 30.)

continued on page 31

Tadalafil for BPH

continued from page 28

Sebastianelli A, Spatafora P, Frizzi J, et al. Tadalafil 5 mg Alone or in Combination with Tamsulosin 0.4 mg for the Management of Men with Lower Urinary Tract Symptoms and Erectile Dysfunction: Results of a Prospective Observational Trial. *Journal of Clinical Medicine* 2019;8(8):1126. PMID: 31362410.

Sebastianelli A, Spatafora P, Morselli S, et al. Tadalafil Alone or in Combination with Tamsulosin for the Management for LUTS/BPH and ED. *Current Urological Reports* 2020;21(12):56. PMID: 33108544.

Singh I, Aravind TK, Gupta S. Efficacy and Safety of Tadalafil vs Tamsulosin in Lower Urinary Tract Symptoms (LUTS) as a Result of Benign Prostate Hyperplasia (BHP)—Open Label Randomised Controlled Study. *International Journal of Clinical Practice* 2020;74(8):e13530. PMID: 32542854.

Takahashi R, Sumino Y, Miyazato M, et al. Tadalafil Improves Nocturia and Nocturia-Related Quality of Life in Patients with Benign Prostatic Hyperplasia (KYU-PRO Study). *Urology International* 2020;104(7–8):587–93. PMID: 32485724.

Antimuscarinics for overactive bladder in men with BPH

Albisinni S, Biaou I, Marcelis Q, et al. New Medical Treatments for Lower Urinary Tract Symptoms Due to Benign Prostatic Hyperplasia and Future Perspectives. *BMC Urology* 2016;16(1):58. PMID: 27629059.

Dahm P, Brasure M, MacDonald R, et al. Comparative Effectiveness of Newer Medications for Lower Urinary Tract Symptoms Attributed to Benign Prostatic Hyperplasia: A Systematic Review and Meta-Analysis. *European Urology* 2017;71(4)570–81. PMID: 27717522.

Drake MJ, Bowditch S, Arbe E, et al. A Retrospective Study of Treatment Persistence and Adherence to α-Blocker plus Antimuscarinic Combination Therapies, in Men with LUTS/BPH in the Netherlands. *BMC Urology* 2017;17(1)36. PMID: 28532455.

PubMed See page 120.

Table 3. BPH procedures compared

Procedure	What's involved	Success rates	Side effects
Transurethral resection of the prostate (TURP)	Performed in operating room. Requires general or spinal anesthesia. May require one to two days in the hospital, with catheter inserted to enable urination for one to three days. Heavy physical activity may be restricted for two weeks or more to prevent bleeding. Full recovery may take four to six weeks.	Provides symptom relief in at least 85%–90% of men treated.	May cause erectile dysfunction or retrograde ejaculation. Blood loss, urinary incontinence, infections, and complications from anesthesia are uncommon but do occur.
Photoselective vaporization of the prostate (PVP or GreenLight)	Most patients treated in outpatient setting. Catheter usually in place overnight. Patients can resume light activity within two to three days and vigorous activity in four to six weeks.	Provides symptom relief similar to TURP.	Ejaculatory problems similar to TURP. Less bleeding than TURP. Urinary frequency or urgency in first month.
Holmium laser enucleation of the prostate (HoLEP)	Performed in operating room. Requires general anesthesia. Overnight catheter may be needed. Heavy physical activity restricted for three to four weeks.	Provides symptom relief similar to TURP. The only BPH surgical procedure endorsed by the American Urological Association for all prostate sizes.	Short-term bleeding, urinary incontinence, infections, ejaculatory problems similar to TURP.
Thulium laser enucleation of the prostate	Performed in a hospital. Most patients go home the day of their surgery.	Limited data suggest symptom relief is similar to HoLEP.	Ejaculatory problems similar to TURP. In rare cases may cause bleeding, urinary incontinence, and infection.
Transurethral microwave thermotherapy (TUMT)	Performed on outpatient basis in a doctor's office. Anesthesia not needed, though pain medication and sedatives may be necessary. Catheter needed for several days.	More effective than medication but less effective than TURP.	Frequent or uncomfortable urination that can last for several weeks. Risk of reoperation is greater than with TURP. Low risk of retrograde ejaculation.
Transurethral electrovapor-ization of the prostate (TUEVP or TVP)	Overnight hospital stay. Catheter needed for one to two days.	As effective as TURP at relieving symptoms and improving urine flow.	Likelihood of urinary retention is greater than with TURP. Risk of reoperation is greater than with TURP. Some urinary side effects, such as blood in the urine and irritation when urinating, that can last for a few weeks. Higher risk of retrograde ejaculation.
Transurethral needle ablation of the prostate (TUNA)	Done on an outpatient basis. May need local anesthesia. Catheter usually not needed.	More effective than medication but less effective than TURP.	Patients may need additional treatments. Erectile dysfunction and urinary incontinence less common than with TURP.
Transurethral incision of the prostate (TUIP)	Requires regional or general anesthesia. Hospital stay is typically one to three days. Usually reserved for men with a small prostate.	About 80% of patients report an improvement in urinary symptoms.	Likelihood of urinary retention and risk of reoperation greater than with TURP.
Prostatic urethral lift (UroLift)	Performed in outpatient setting under local or general anesthesia. Approximately 95% of treated men return home the same day without a catheter. Heavy physical activity may be restricted for two weeks or more to prevent bleeding.	Provides symptom relief similar to TURP.	Transient blood in urine and burning sensations while urinating that clear up in two to three days.
Water vapor thermal therapy (Rezum)	Performed in a doctor's office or outpatient facility under local anesthesia. Catheter used for several days. Light exercise allowed within a few days, strenuous exercise within two weeks.	More effective than medication but less effective than TURP.	Does not cause erectile dysfunction. Side effects, including painful urination, blood in urine or semen, frequent urination, or inability to empty the bladder completely, generally resolve within three weeks.

Figure 3. Transurethral resection of the prostate (TURP)

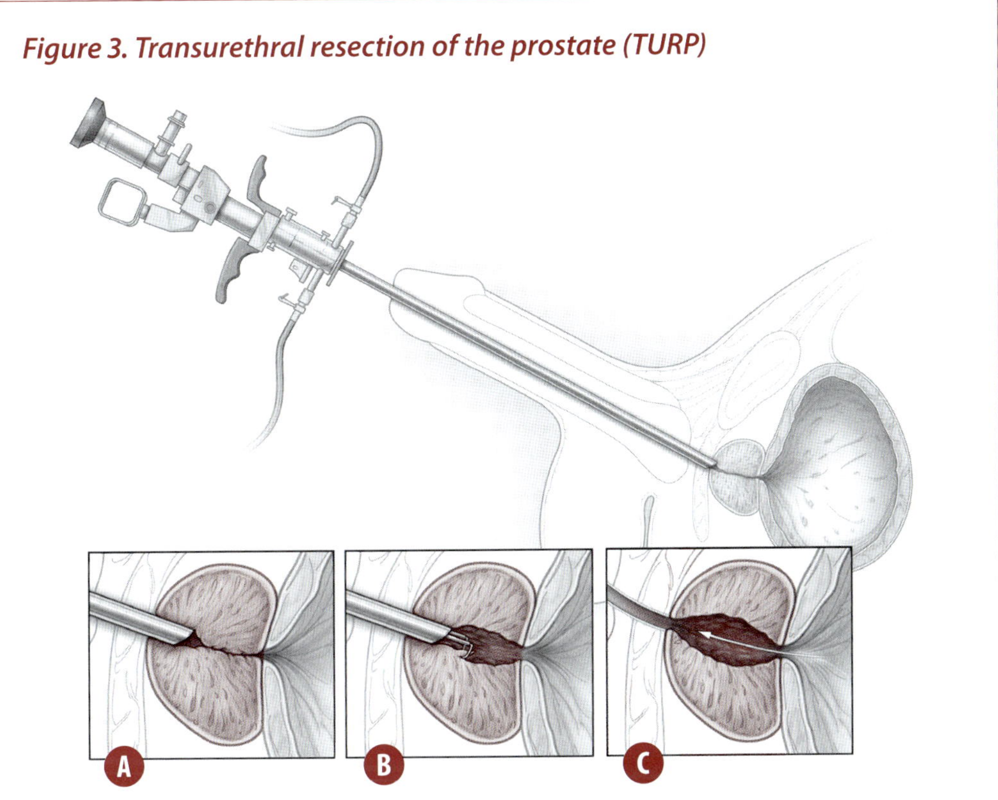

During transurethral resection of the prostate (TURP), the surgeon inserts a thin tube called a resectoscope into the urethra and threads it up into the enlarged prostate (**A**). The resectoscope contains a tiny camera, which enables the surgeon to view the gland throughout the operation, as well as an electrical loop. The surgeon uses the loop to chip away at overgrown prostate tissue that's pressing on the urethra and narrowing it (**B**). After the procedure, the enlarged passageway allows urine to flow more easily (**C**).

continued from page 29

Transurethral resection of the prostate (TURP). TURP, often inelegantly referred to as the "roto-rooter" technique, is an incision-free surgical procedure that cuts away excess prostate tissue with an electrical loop (see Figure 3, above). The removed tissues can then be examined by a pathologist to see if any cancer is present. TURP remains the most common form of prostate surgery and is usually more successful than medication. It relieves urinary obstruction in at least 85% to 90% of men, and the improvement usually lasts. However, urinary problems can recur if the prostate tissue grows back. Not surprisingly, the younger you are, the more likely it is that you'll eventually need another treatment.

The hourlong procedure takes place in an operating room under general or spinal anesthesia, given just before the operation begins. You may spend one to two days recovering in the hospital. While recovering, you will urinate through a catheter inserted into the bladder through the penis. Once home, you may have to restrict heavy physical activity for two weeks or more to prevent bleeding.

About two-thirds of the men who have TURP experience retrograde ejaculation, in which semen travels backward into the bladder when they ejaculate. The semen released is soon flushed out of the body in urine. Retrograde ejaculation has no effect on orgasm sensation. However, it can make it more difficult to father children.

Between 5% and 10% of TURP patients experience serious complications such as blood loss, impotence, urinary incontinence, infections, and complications related to the anesthesia. The risk of these complications needs to be considered when choosing treatment options. Still, TURP remains the standard treatment for BPH—a treatment with a long, proven track record.

About 2% of men who have the procedure develop TURP syndrome in the hospital. This short-lived state is marked by symptoms such as confusion, nausea, vomiting, high blood pressure, and visual distortions. The syndrome—often shortened to TUR syndrome—develops as a complication of absorption of the irrigation fluid used to keep the surgical area clean during TURP.

A safer alternative is saline (salt water) solution used in combination with a special surgical instrument called a coaxial continuous-flow bipolar resectoscope. A 2017 study found that the bipolar procedure performed with saline solution was less likely than the traditional monopolar procedure to cause TURP syndrome and the formation of blood clots that block the flow of urine out of the bladder. That's because performing the procedure this way results in less absorption of the fluids that cause TURP syndrome. In other studies, men also needed less time with a catheter and had shorter hospital stays after the bipolar procedure, and research has detected no difference between the two methods in terms of sexual side effects and other complications. (For references, see "Bipolar vs. monopolar TURP," above left.)

Photoselective vaporization of the prostate (PVP, or GreenLight). While TURP remains the mainstay of the surgical treatments for BPH, laser surgery is becoming increasingly popular. With this approach, excess prostate tissue is destroyed by laser energy, and the remnants are excreted in urine. Typically, patients go home the same day as laser surgery, even if the procedure is performed at a hospital. Studies increasingly show little to no difference between surgery and laser treatments when it comes to resolving urinary symptoms in men with BPH. But there are short-term differences: TURP is associated with more frequent blood transfusions, longer hospital stays, longer catheterization times, and more frequent—but still very rare—postoperative complications such as pneumonia and septic shock.

Results from a 2017 study showed that TURP-treated men had more pain after surgery and a slower return to normal life than men treated with photoselective vaporization of the prostate (PVP), one common type of laser procedure. On the flip side, men who've had TURP score better on measures of symptom control and quality of life after five years, while men who've had PVP are more likely to need a repeat procedure to address recurring urinary symptoms, according to a 2021 review of 12 studies. This may occur if the laser is too weak to remove enough prostate tissue. As more powerful lasers have come into wider use, however, success rates of TURP and PVP are becoming comparable. (For references, see "PVP laser procedure for BPH," at left.)

To perform PVP, the surgeon begins by guiding a thin, flexible optic fiber through the urethra to the prostate. This fiber conducts the laser light to the target area of the prostate. Most laser procedures involve focusing the energy of the laser so it destroys

Bipolar vs. monopolar TURP

Al-Rawashdah SF, Pastore AL, Salhi YA, et al. Prospective Randomized Study Comparing Monopolar with Bipolar Transurethral Resection of Prostate in Benign Prostatic Obstruction: 36-Month Outcomes. *World Journal of Urology* 2017;35(10):1595–601. PMID: 28243790.

Egui Rojo MA, Redón Gálvez L, Álvarez Ardura M, et al. Comparison of Monopoloar Versus Bipolar Transurethral Resection of the Prostate: Evaluation of the Impact on Sexual Function. *Revista Internacional de Andrología* 2020;18(2):43–49. PMID: 30612924.

Kumar BN, Srivastava A, Sinha T. Urethral Stricture After Bipolar Transurethral Resection of Prostate—Truth vs Hype: A Randomized Controlled Trial. *Indian Journal of Urology* 2019;35(1):41–47. PMID: 30692723.

PVP laser procedure for BPH

Bachmann A, Tubaro A, Barber N, et al. A European Multicenter Randomized Noninferiority Trial Comparing 180 W GreenLight XPS Laser Vaporization and Transurethral Resection of the Prostate for the Treatment of Benign Prostatic Obstruction: 12-Month Results of the GOLIATH study. *Journal of Urology* 2015;193(2):570–78. PMID: 25219699.

Castellani D, Pirola GM, Rubilotta E, et al. GreenLight Laser Photovaporization versus Transurethral Resection of the Prostate: A Systematic Review and Meta-Analysis. *Research and Reports in Urology* 2021;13:263–71. PMID: 34295844.

Cimino S, Voce S, Palmieri F, et al. Transurethral Resection of the Prostate (TURP) vs GreenLight Photoselective Vaporization of Benign Prostatic Hyperplasia: Analysis of BPH6 Outcomes After 1 Year of Follow-Up. *International Journal of Impotence Research* 2017;29(6):240–43. PMID: 28814812.

Ghobrial FK, Shoma A, Elshal AM, et al. A Randomized Trial Comparing Bipolar Transurethral Vaporization of the Prostate with Greenlight Laser (xps-180 watt) Photoselective Vaporization of the Prostate for Treatment of Small to Moderate Benign Prostatic Obstruction: Outcomes After 2 Years. *BJU International* 2020;125(1):144–52. PMID: 31621175.

continued on page 33

the overgrown tissue. However, this destruction of tissue gives laser procedures a significant disadvantage: prostate tissue destroyed with a laser can't be checked for cancer, whereas TURP yields tissue samples that a pathologist can examine.

Various kinds of lasers are used in procedures to treat BPH. The KTP (which stands for potassium-titanyl-phosphate) laser, also known as GreenLight, is used in the PVP procedure. It produces a visible green light that is selectively absorbed by hemoglobin-rich prostate tissue. The trapped energy produces vapor bubbles that destroy the tissue from within. This procedure also cauterizes blood vessels to reduce bleeding. One of the chief advantages of PVP is that patients on blood-thinning medications like warfarin can have the procedure and still take their medications.

The KTP lasers that surgeons use today are two or even three times more powerful than the lasers used 10 years ago, when PVP was developed. The more powerful lasers mean surgeons can work faster, so operating times are shorter, and they also remove tissue more effectively, reducing the likelihood men will need a repeat procedure.

Holmium laser enucleation of the prostate (HoLEP). Other lasers used to treat BPH include the holmium and thulium lasers. Both are used to cut away prostate tissue, a procedure called enucleation. HoLEP is the only BPH surgical procedure endorsed by the American Urological Association (AUA) for all prostate sizes, leading some researchers to contend that HoLEP should now be regarded as the new gold standard for BPH surgery.

A 2019 review article concluded that HoLEP is at least as effective as TURP for reducing BPH symptoms, with benefits potentially lasting more than 10 years. Its advantages included less need for blood transfusion and also shorter catheterization and hospital stays. Another paper, published in 2021, found the procedure was effec-

PVP laser procedure for BPH

continued from page 32

Malik RD, Wang CE, Lapin B, et al. Comparison of Patients Undergoing Laser Vaporization of the Prostate Versus TURP Using the ACS-NSQIP Database. *Prostate Cancer and Prostatic Diseases* 2015;18(1):18–24. PMID: 25311768.

Sandhu JS, Leong LY, Das AK. Photoselective Vaporization of the Prostate: Application, Outcomes, and Safety. *Canadian Journal of Urology* 2019;26(4S1):8–12. PMID: 31481143.

PubMed See page 120.

Figure 4. Photoselective vaporization of the prostate (PVP)

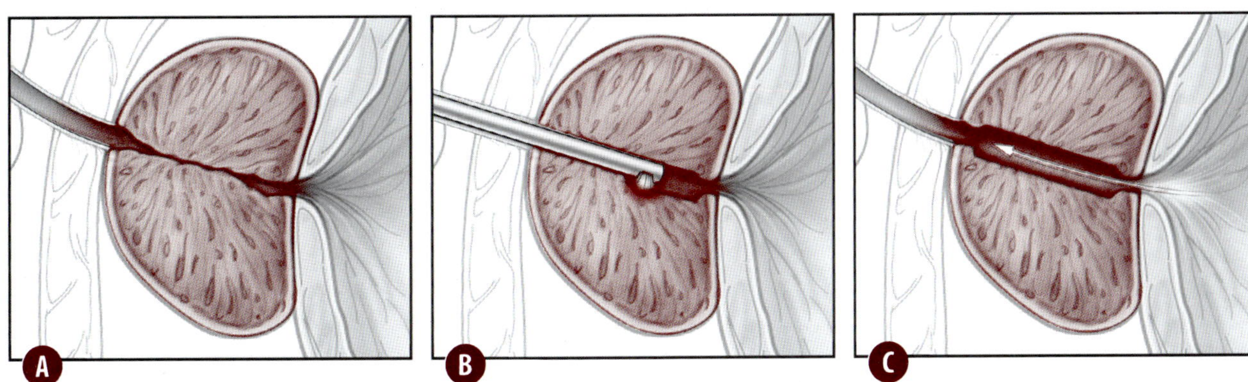

When an enlarged prostate obstructs urine flow (**A**), a laser technique may be used instead of TURP. During photoselective vaporization of the prostate (PVP), also called the GreenLight procedure, the surgeon threads a thin tube called a cystoscope through the urethra into the enlarged prostate. The surgeon then passes a fiber optic device through the cystoscope to generate high-intensity pulses of light, which simultaneously vaporize the obstructing tissue and cauterize it to reduce bleeding (**B**). This creates an enlarged, uniform channel through which urine can flow (**C**).

tive for very large prostates, weighing more than 200 grams, which have traditionally posed a challenge for surgeons. Still, not all surgeons are comfortable using HoLEP for very large prostates. (For references, see "Holmium and thulium laser procedures for BPH," at left.)

Thulium laser enucleation of the prostate. Thulium laser enucleation is similar to HoLEP. The main difference is that the holmium approach uses pulsed laser energy, while the thulium procedure uses continuous laser energy. The thulium method may result in less blood loss during surgery. A 2016 study concluded that thulium laser enucleation effectively reduced urinary symptoms in 177 treated patients without affecting erectile function (although some patients did have ejaculation problems). A 2020 study involving 116 men found that the holmium and thulium procedures relieved urinary symptoms equally well during the 18-month study period. (For references, see "Holmium and thulium laser procedures for BPH," at left.)

Updated BPH treatment guidelines published by the AUA in 2020 stated that either HoLEP or the thulium method can be considered for treating enlarged prostates, depending on the surgeon's own experience. (For reference, see "BPH guidelines," page 35.)

Transurethral microwave thermotherapy (TUMT). Sometimes referred to as "heat therapy," TUMT uses microwaves to destroy prostate tissue. The doctor guides a thin catheter carrying a miniature microwave generator through the urethra to the prostate. The purpose is the same as with many of the other techniques: to remove prostate tissue that is squeezing the urethra. How much microwaved heat is used varies, but surgeons can dial it up to between 140° F and 170° F. A cooling jacket around the microwave generator protects the urethra, and a heat sensor in a rectal probe helps make sure the temperature doesn't get too high. A review published in 2021 reported that while TUMT provides symptom relief comparable to TURP in the short run, along with fewer complications and fewer problems with sexual dysfunction, it is also more likely to require repeat treatment. (For reference, see "TUMT for BPH," page 35.)

Transurethral electrovaporization of the prostate (TUEVP or TVP). Like TURP, TUEVP involves threading the resectoscope up through the urethra. But instead of cutting tissue away with a wire loop, the surgeon heats and vaporizes tissue using a ball-shaped electrode. The electrode also cauterizes (seals off) blood vessels in the treated area to minimize bleeding. A 2020 study with 58 patients reported that TUEVP and PVP achieved similar symptom improvements that were still holding up at two years. (For reference, see "PVP laser procedure for BPH," page 32.)

Transurethral needle ablation (TUNA). TUNA is a thermal approach that uses low-level radio waves delivered through twin needles to heat and kill obstructing prostate cells. Shields are used to protect the urethra from damage. The treatment can improve symptoms, quality of life, and urine flow with little risk of sexual side effects, but TURP typically generates better results for urinary function.

Transurethral incision of the prostate (TUIP). TUIP also involves inserting an instrument into the prostate via the penis. But instead of cutting away or vaporizing excess tissue, the surgeon makes one or more lengthwise incisions in the prostate at

Holmium and thulium laser procedures for BPH

Das AK, Teplitsky S, Humphreys MR. Holmium Laser Enucleation of the Prostate (HoLEP): A Review and Update. *Canadian Journal of Urology* 2019;26(4S1):13–19. PMID: 31481144.

Elshal AM, Elkoushy MA, El-Nahas AR, et al. GreenLight Laser (XPS) Photoselective Vapo-Enucleation Versus Holmium Laser Enucleation of the Prostate for the Treatment of Symptomatic Benign Prostatic Hyperplasia: A Randomized Controlled Study. *Journal of Urology* 2015;193(3):927–34. PMID: 25261801.

Pirola GM, Saredi G, Codas Duarte R, et al. Holmium Laser Versus Thulium Laser Enucleation of the Prostate: A Matched-Pair Analysis from Two Centers. *Therapeutic Advances in Urology* 2018;10(8):223–33. PMID: 30034541.

Romero-Otero J, Garcia-Gomez B, Garcia-Gonzalez L, et al. Critical Analysis of a Multicentric Experience with Holmium Laser Enucleation of the Prostate for Benign Prostatic Hyperplasia: Outcomes and Complications of 10 Years of Routine Clinical Practice. *BJU International* 2020;126(1):177–82. PMID: 32020749.

Saredi T, Pacchetti A, Pirola GM, et al. Impact of Thulium Laser Enucleation of the Prostate on Erectile, Ejaculatory and Urinary Functions. *Urologia Internationalis* 2016;97(4):397–401. PMID: 27463971.

Shvero A, Calio B, Humphreys MR, et al. HoLEP: The New Gold Standard for Surgical Treatment of Benign Prostatic Hyperplasia. *Canadian Journal of Urology* 2021;28(S2): 6–10. PMID: 34453422.

Zell MA, Haidar AM, Navaratnam A, et al. Holmium Laser Enucleation of the Prostate for Very Large Benign Prostatic Hyperplasia (≥ 200 cc). *World Journal of Urology* 2021;39(1):129–34. PMID: 32206890.

Zhang J, Ou Z, Xiaobo Z, et al. Holmium Laser Enucleation of the Prostate vs Thulium Laser Enucleation of the Prostate for the Treatment of Large-Volume Prostates > 80 ml: 18-Month Followup Results. *World Journal of Urology* 2020;38(6):1555–62. PMID: 31502032.

the site of the urethral constriction. This opens the urethral passage, relieving pressure on the urethra and improving urine flow.

Prostatic urethral lift. The prostatic urethral lift procedure involves pulling back the lobes of the prostate gland so they no longer impinge on the urethra. The "lifts" are small lengths of monofilament, permanently implanted in the gland. In 2013, the FDA approved a device called the UroLift system for prostates 80 grams or under that allows doctors to insert the device directly into the urethra, so it functions much like a prostatic urethral stent (below).

A 2017 study with more than 200 patients found that the urethral lift provided improvements in BPH symptoms and quality of life that held up five years after treatment. During that study, the urethral lift improved urinary symptom scores by 36% and quality-of-life measures by 40%, while preserving normal erectile and ejaculatory function. Only 13.6% of the men required additional treatment within five years, meaning that about 86% of them avoided retreatment. A 2020 review of 11 studies involving 2,016 patients determined that the retreatment rate after three years of follow-up averaged 10.7%. While the AUA guidelines generally limit the procedure to men with prostate sizes of no more than 80 grams, a 2019 study found that the procedure provided rapid symptom relief while preserving sexual function for two years in 86 men with prostates weighing up to 111 grams. (For references, see "Prostatic urethral lift," at right.)

Water vapor thermal therapy (Rezum). Pronounced "resume," this is a more recent noninvasive procedure for BPH. Patients can be treated in a doctor's office, under local anesthesia and sometimes a nerve block to minimize pain. To perform the procedure, the doctor inserts a thin hollow tube, called a scope, through the penis into the prostate. The scope delivers nine-second blasts of steam that kill prostate cells, causing the enlarged tissues to shrink over time, widening the urethral channel so that the man can urinate normally. Procedure-related side effects, including urine retention and painful urination, typically resolve within three weeks.

A 2020 review of four studies with a combined total of 514 men found that Rezum-treated men still had significant improvements in urinary functioning four years after treatment—without sexual side effects. Roughly 7% of the treated men had to have a repeat surgery. (For references, see "Rezum for BPH," below right.)

The FDA hasn't cleared Rezum for prostates weighing more than 80 grams, so the procedure isn't available to men with the largest prostates.

Other BPH treatments

A variety of other treatments are in use. They aren't available everywhere. Some aren't covered by insurance. Others may be available only as part of a clinical trial.

Prostatic urethral stents. A prostatic urethral stent is a small, springlike mesh cylinder. The doctor inserts the stent through the penis and, after positioning it in the narrowed area of the urethra, releases it to widen the channel, relieving pressure from the prostate tissue and permitting easier urination. This quick procedure requires only local or spinal anesthesia, involves no loss of blood, and is often done in an outpatient surgical center.

BPH guidelines

Parsons JK, Dahm P, Koller TS, et al. Surgical Management of Lower Urinary Tract Symptoms Attributed to Benign Prostatic Hyperplasia: AUA Guideline Amendment 2020. *Journal of Urology* 2020;204(4):799–804. PMID: 32698710.

TUMT for BPH

Franco JVA, Garegnani L, Escobar Liquitay CM, et al. Transurethral Microwave Thermotherapy for Benign Prostatic Hyperplasia: An Updated Cochrane Review. *World Journal of Men's Health* 2022;40(1):127–38. PMID: 34448377.

Prostatic urethral lift

Miller LE, Chughtai B, Dornbier RA, et al. Surgical Reintervention Rate After Prostatic Urethral Lift: Systematic Review and Meta-Analysis Involving Over 2,000 Patients. *Journal of Urology* 2020;204(5):1019–26. PMID: 32396049.

Roehrborn CG, Barkin J, Gange SN, et al. Five-Year Results of the Prospective Randomized Controlled Prostatic Urethral L.I.F.T. Study. *Canadian Journal of Urology* 2017;24(3):8802–13. PMID: 28646935.

Rukstalis D, Grier D, Stroup SP, et al. Prostatic Urethral Lift (PUL) for Obstructive Median Lobes: 12 Month Results of the MedLift Study. *Prostate Cancer and Prostatic Diseases* 2019;22(3):411–19. PMID: 30542055.

Sievert KD, Schonthaler M, Berges R, et al. Minimally Invasive Prostatic Urethral Lift (PUL) Efficacious in TURP Candidates: A Multicenter German Evaluation After 2 Years. *World Journal of Urology* 2019;37(7):1353–60. PMID: 30283994.

Rezum for BPH

Green Z, Westwood J, Somani BK. What's New in Rezum: A Transurethral Water Vapour Therapy for BPH. *Current Urology Reports* 2019;20(7):39. PMID: 31152253.

Miller LE, Chughtai B, McVary K, et al. Water Vapor Thermal Therapy for Lower Urinary Tract Symptoms Secondary to Benign Prostatic Hyperplasia: Systematic Review and Meta-Analysis. *Medicine (Baltimore)* 2020;99(30):e21365. PMID: 32791742.

PubMed See page 120.

Aquablation

Gilling P, Barber N, Bidair M, et al. Three-Year Outcomes After Aquablation Therapy Compared to TURP: Results from a Blinded Randomized Trial. *Canadian Journal of Urology* 2020;27(1):10072–79. PMID: 32065861.

Misrai V, Rijo E, Zorn KC, et al. Waterjet Ablation Therapy for Treating Benign Prostatic Obstruction in Patients with Small- to Medium-Size Glands: 12-Month Results of the First French Aquablation Clinical Registry. *European Urology* 2019;76(5):667–75. PMID: 31281024.

Roehrborn CG, Teplitzky S, Das AK. Aquablation of the Prostate: A Review and Update. *Canadian Journal of Urology* 2019;26(4S1):20–24. PMID: 31481145.

Zorn K, Bidair M, Bhojani N, et al. Aquablation for Benign Prostatic Hyperplasia in Large Prostates (80–150cc): 3-Year Results. Presented at the 2021 Annual Meeting of the American Urological Association. Abstract No. PD18–06.

Prostatic artery embolization

Abt D, Hechelhammer L, Müllhaupt G, et al. Comparison of Prostatic Artery Embolization (PAE) Versus Transurethral Resection of the Prostate (TURP) for Benign Prostatic Hyperplasia: Randomised, Open Label, Non-Inferiority Trial. *BMJ* 2018;361:k2338. PMID: 29921613.

Srinivasan A, Wang R. An Update on Minimally Invasive Surgery for Benign Prostatic Hyperplasia: Techniques, Risks, and Efficacy. *World Journal of Men's Health* 2020;38(4):402–11. PMID: 31496146.

Xiang P, Guan D, Du Z, et al. Efficacy and Safety of Prostatic Artery Embolization for Benign Prostatic Hyperplasia: A Systematic Review and Meta-Analysis of Randomized Controlled Trials. *European Radiology* 2021;31(7):4929–46. PMID: 33449181.

PubMed See page 120.

Prostatic urethral stents are most often used in elderly men who have severe prostate enlargement and whose overall health is poor, meaning more involved surgery would be risky. In many cases, urinary obstruction gradually returns after the placement of the stents, and additional procedures may be required in some instances.

Aquablation. This new robotic-assisted technique destroys prostate tissue with jets of highly pressurized saline delivered under guidance from ultrasound. The robotic system ensures that only tissues mapped by ultrasound are removed. After the procedure, doctors cauterize the area to limit bleeding. Aquablation requires further investigation to confirm its effectiveness over time, but studies are encouraging.

In 2020, researchers published findings from a clinical trial comparing aquablation with TURP in 181 men, whose prostates weighed 30 to 80 grams and whose BPH symptoms were moderate to severe. Symptom relief was nearly identical even after three years of follow-up, and the aquablation-treated men retained their ability to ejaculate normally. Men with larger prostate glands of up to 150 grams also achieved substantial symptom relief from aquablation at three years, according to a study presented in 2021. Procedures performed on the larger prostates were associated with higher rates of low-grade complications, including blood loss during surgery. (For references, see "Aquablation," above left.)

Prostatic artery embolization (PAE). In this procedure, a radiologist inserts a catheter into the femoral artery and guides it toward the prostate. After it's positioned in the artery supplying blood to the prostate, the catheter is used to deliver microscopic spheres that block blood flow. This causes the prostate to shrink. This approach has been used in the United States only since 2017, and it is still not widely available. Some experts say that PAE poses lesser risks of long-term side effects (such as retrograde ejaculation, incontinence, or sexual dysfunction) compared with other procedures.

A 2018 paper comparing PAE with monopolar TURP reported fewer complications from PAE at 12 weeks, along with less blood loss, shorter catheterization, and briefer hospital stays. But functional outcomes—such as improved urinary flow rates and the ability to empty the bladder better—favored TURP, and some studies have found failure rates of up to 19% (meaning that urinary symptoms worsen again) within a year, according to a 2020 review article. A 2021 review of 11 published articles reported no significant difference between TURP and PAE in terms of symptom improvements at two years. However, this represents very short follow-up, and more data are needed to confirm long-term benefits from PAE and to see how well it compares with other procedures. As of 2021, the AUA was not recommending PAE outside of clinical trials. (For references, see "Prostatic artery embolization," at left.)

Dr. Garnick cautions that in rare instances, PAE can cause blood clots to accumulate in the bladder, a dangerous complication that requires surgery. The 2020 AUA guidelines state that because the risk/benefit ratio with PAE remains unclear, it should be done only as part of a clinical trial. (For reference, see "BPH guidelines," page 35.)

Prostate cancer

What you need to know at every stage of the disease

Prostate cancer is the second most commonly diagnosed cancer in men in the United States, and the second leading cause of cancer death among men (after lung cancer). The American Cancer Society (ACS) estimates that 248,530 American men were diagnosed with the disease in 2020, and 34,130 died of it—although definitive numbers won't be available for a couple of years, since it takes time for scientists to gather and analyze data. According to the ACS, the 10-year survival rate for all stages combined is 98%, and the 15-year survival rate is 96%.

Most men diagnosed with prostate cancer learn they have the disease after a blood test finds abnormal levels of prostate-specific antigen (PSA)—a protein that prostate cancer cells release in high amounts—or after a digital rectal exam (DRE) reveals an enlarged or irregular prostate, followed by a biopsy that confirms cancer. Very few men are diagnosed after experiencing symptoms, such as difficulties with urination, or evidence that the cancer may have spread, as indicated by bone or back pain.

Nine out of every 10 cases of prostate cancer these days are detected at the local or regional stage (see "Prostate cancer terminology," page 38). When the disease is discovered at these early stages, the five-year survival rate approaches 100%.

What causes prostate cancer?

No one knows precisely what causes prostate cancer. But that doesn't mean it's a total mystery, either. Genetic defects play a role in the development of any cancer, as do environmental carcinogens that cause DNA damage. In some instances, the defects are inherited, meaning that they affect DNA in the parent's sperm or egg cells (which are also called germ cells) and carry through into the developing baby. These inherited (germline) defects will be present in every cell of a man's body, but their cancer-causing effects tend to be selective for specific organs, including the prostate.

For example, the same germline defects in the BRCA1 and BRCA2 genes that boost the risk of breast and ovarian cancer in women have also been linked to aggressive, hard-to-treat prostate cancers that affect younger men. BRCA genes ordinarily repair DNA damage. When those genes are defective, DNA damage can accumulate inside cells that, in turn, grow abnormally and form tumors. Roughly a quarter of all men who have aggressive prostate cancer have defects in one or both of these genes, but most commonly in BRCA2 alone. DNA repair defects aren't limited to just BRCA: investigators have found more than 80 inherited mutations affecting as many as 16 different DNA repair genes that could potentially be involved in prostate cancer, and research published in 2019 found that men with aggressive prostate cancer are three times more likely to have defective DNA repair genes than men whose tumors are growing more slowly.

Genes and prostate cancer

Antonarakis ES, Vehlo PI, Fu W, et al. CDK12-Altered Prostate Cancer: Clinical Features and Therapeutic Outcomes to Standard Systemic Therapies, Poly (ADP-Ribose) Polymerase Inhibitors, and PD-1 Inhibitors. *JCO Precison Oncology* 2020;4:370–81. PMID: 32462107.

Cheng HH, Sokolova AO, Schaeffer EM, et al. Germline and Somatic Mutations in Prostate Cancer for the Clinician. *Journal of the National Comprehensive Cancer Network* 2019;17(5):515–21. PMID: 31085765.

Darst BF, Dadaev T, Saunders E, et al. Germline Sequencing DNA Repair Genes in 5,545 Men with Aggressive and Non-aggressive Prostate Cancer. *Journal of the National Cancer Institute* 2020;2021;113(5):616–25. PMID: 32853339.

Horak P, Weischenfeldt J, von Amsberg G, et al. Response to Olaparib in a PALB2 Germline Mutated Prostate Cancer and Genetic Events Associated with Resistance. *Case Reports* 2019;5(2):a003657. PMID: 30833416.

Marshall CH, Fu W, Wang H, et al. Prevalence of DNA Repair Gene Mutations in Localized Prostate Cancer According to Clinical And Pathologic Features: Association of Gleason Score and Tumor Stage. *Prostate Cancer and Prostatic Diseases* 2019;22(1):59–65. PMID: 30171229.

continued on page 39

Other germline genetic defects implicated in prostate cancer occur in the ATM gene (which helps regulate cell growth), in the HOXB13 gene (which plays a role in prostate development), in the PALB2 gene (which coordinates with BRCA2 in the DNA damage response), in the CDK12 gene (which helps to stabilize the cell genome), and in so-called mismatch repair genes (which repair DNA errors that allow cancer cells to survive for unusually long durations and to resist chemotherapy). Men with advanced prostate cancer can also have gene mutations that boost their sensitivity to testosterone, making their prostate cancer cells grow more aggressively. If they have metastatic cancer and defects in a gene called CHEK2, they are not as likely to respond to hormonal treatments that aim to blunt testosterone's effects. Fortunately, as many as 90% of the gene defects that have been found so far in advanced prostate cancer can be targeted with existing drugs or drugs that are now in clinical trials. (For references, see "Genes and prostate cancer," at left.)

Doctors screen for germline mutations in saliva, urine, and blood samples. But other genetic defects, which are not inherited, can develop if chemicals, radiation, or inflammation alter DNA. These somatic mutations, as they are known, are found only in the cells descending from the cell that was originally mutated, and some of them may cause prostate cancer. Doctors look for them in tumor samples.

Risk factors

Risk factors are sometimes confused with causes. Risk factors are characteristics or conditions that increase the odds of getting a disease. So while the causes of most prostate cancers remain elusive, innumerable studies have identified risk factors. Here are some of them.

Prostate cancer terminology

Experts classify prostate cancer according to how far it has spread and how it responds to treatment.

Localized prostate cancer is contained within the prostate gland. It is typically treated with surgery or radiation and has the most favorable prognosis.

Regionally advanced prostate cancer has spread out of the prostate into nearby tissues. The treatment is similar to that used for localized cancer and in some instances includes androgen deprivation therapy (ADT), which induces a form of chemical castration that blocks the production of testosterone and therefore testosterone's growth-promoting effects on prostate cancer cells. This will ideally eliminate the cancer or slow its growth.

Biochemical recurrence refers to a rise in PSA levels following initial treatment with surgery, radiation, or both, without any metastases that are visible on imaging scans. This suggests that cancer cells lurk unseen somewhere in the body.

- If subsequent treatment with ADT causes the PSA levels to fall, indicating that hormonal therapy is working, the condition is called **nonmetastatic castration-sensitive prostate cancer (nmCSPC)**.
- If PSA levels continue to climb despite the use of ADT, indicating that hormonal therapy is not working, the condition is called **nonmetastatic castration-resistant prostate cancer (nmCRPC)**. In recent years, newer, more potent forms of ADT have become available for treating this condition. These treatments suppress testosterone in ways that differ from the frontline forms of ADT given initially.

Metastatic castration-sensitive prostate cancer (mCSPC) produces metastases that show up on imaging scans, and it responds to frontline ADT.

Metastatic castration-resistant prostate cancer (mCRPC) produces metastases that show up on imaging scans, and it has become unresponsive to frontline ADT.

Oligometastatic prostate cancer is defined by the presence of five or fewer metastatic tumors that appear on imaging.

Age. The risk of prostate cancer increases with age. The disease rarely occurs among men under 40. About 90% of cases are diagnosed in men over age 55, and the median age for diagnosis is 66, according to the National Cancer Institute's Surveillance, Epidemiology, and End Results (SEER) data. The number of cases diagnosed tapers off in men ages 75 and older, partly because men in that age group aren't screened as often.

Family history. Prostate cancer runs in families. A man who has a father or brother with prostate cancer is two to three times more likely to have prostate cancer—or to develop the disease in the future—than a man with no first-degree male relatives with the disease. If two or more first-degree relatives have a prostate cancer history, the risk is five to 10 times greater than for the man with no affected first-degree relatives. The age at which relatives are diagnosed also has some bearing on the risk calculations. Diagnosis before age 60 increases the risk, probably because early-onset prostate cancer is more likely to be caused by inherited mutations.

Race. Black men have the highest prostate cancer incidence and death rates of any group in the United States. The incidence of prostate cancer among Black men is almost 60% higher than it is among white men (178.3 vs. 105.7 per 100,000 men, according to analysis of cases reported to the National Institutes of Health between 2011 and 2015 that has yet to be updated), and the death rate from the disease for Black men is more than double the rate for their white counterparts. This discrepancy probably reflects multiple factors, including disparities in health care and differences in diet. New research published in 2021 suggests that genetic risk factors may also play a role. The researchers behind this study—which is the largest investigation of prostate cancer genetics conducted so far—gathered data from 200,000 men worldwide. They found 86 new genetic variants that boost the risk for prostate cancer. Those variants were then incorporated into a model showing that those men of African descent have roughly twice the inherited prostate cancer risk than men with European ancestry. (See "Large genetics study shows Blacks at higher risk of prostate cancer," page 10, and "Race and prostate cancer risk," at right.)

Nationality. Prostate cancer incidence varies greatly among countries. The highest rates are in Australia and New Zealand, Western Europe, Canada and the United States, and the Caribbean, while the lowest rates are in south central Asia (Thailand and India) and northern Africa.

Obesity. Obesity seems to increase the risk of developing and dying from aggressive prostate cancer, particularly among men who are overweight during their 50s and 60s. (For references, see "Body weight and prostate cancer risk," at right.) One potential explanation involves insulin, the hormone that enables cells in the body to use energy from glucose and fatty acids in the blood. Excess weight causes people to develop insulin resistance, a condition in which cells become less sensitive to insulin's effects. To compensate for this resistance, their bodies produce higher and higher levels of insulin over time. Insulin is a growth factor, so as the insulin level rises, it may help drive the out-of-control cell growth in cancer directly or through the action of related hormones called insulin-like growth factors.

Genes and prostate cancer

continued from page 38

Na R, Zheng SL, Han M, et al. Germline Mutations in ATM and BRCA1/2 Distinguish Risk for Lethal and Indolent Prostate Cancer and Are Associated with Early Age at Death. *European Urology* 2017;71(5):740–47. PMID: 27989354.

Nicolosi P, Ledet E, Yang S, et al. Prevalence of Germline Variants in Prostate Cancer and Implications for Current Genetic Testing Guidelines. *JAMA Oncology* 2019;5(4):523–28. PMID: 30730552.

Pritchard CC, Mateo J, Walsh MF, et al. Inherited DNA-Repair Gene Mutations in Men with Metastatic Prostate Cancer. *New England Journal of Medicine* 2016;375(5):443–53. PMID: 27433846.

Quigley DA, Dang HX, Zhao SG, et al. Genomic Hallmarks and Structural Variation in Metastatic Prostate Cancer. *Cell* 2018;174(3):758–69. PMID: 30033370.

Velho PI, Lim D, Wang H, et al. Molecular Characterization and Clinical Outcomes of Primary Gleason Pattern 5 Prostate Cancer After Radical Prostatectomy. *JCO Precision Oncology* 2019;3:PO.19.00081. PMID: 31650100.

Wu Y, Yu H, Zheng SL, et al. A Comprehensive Evaluation of CHEK2 Germline Mutations in Men with Prostate Cancer. *Prostate* 2018;78(8):607–15. PMID: 29520813.

Race and prostate cancer risk

Conti DV, Darst BF, Moss LC, et al. Trans-Ancestry Genome-Wide Association Meta-Analysis of Prostate Cancer Identifies New Susceptibility Loci and Informs Genetic Risk Prediction. *Nature Genetics* 2021;53(1):65–75. PMID: 33398198.

Body weight and prostate cancer risk

Genkinger JM, Wu K, Wang M, et al. Measures of Body Fatness and Height in Early and Mid-to-Late Adulthood and Prostate Cancer: Risk and Mortality in the Pooling Project of Prospective Studies of Diet and Cancer. *Annals of Oncology* 2020;31(1):103–14. PMID: 31912782.

Troeschel AN, Hartman TJ, Jacobs EJ, et al. Postdiagnosis Body Mass Index, Weight Change, and Mortality from Prostate Cancer, Cardiovascular Disease, and All Causes Among Survivors of Nonmetastatic Prostate Cancer. *Journal of Clinical Oncology* 2020;38(18):2018–27. PMID: 32250715.

PubMed See page 120.

Diet. Another factor that can increase a person's insulin levels is diet. So-called insulinemic diets that are high in sugary sweets, fried foods, processed snacks, saturated fats, and starchy vegetables also trigger chronic inflammation, which is a risk factor for a number of diseases, including prostate cancer. In 2021, researchers published results from a prospective study with 28 years of follow-up showing that insulinemic and inflammatory dietary patterns boost the risk of aggressive prostate cancer, especially in younger men.

Men who eat a lot of red meat or high-fat dairy products also seem to have a higher risk of developing the disease. Scientists have linked diets high in cholesterol and saturated fat—the type of fat found in fatty beef and cheese—to prostate cancers that are more aggressive, while a 2017 study found that diets rich in fruits, vegetables, legumes, nuts, and fish are protective against aggressive prostate cancers. It is not clear precisely why high-fat diets might boost prostate cancer risk. However, a study with lab mice, published in 2019, suggests that such diets trigger certain genes called oncogenes that push prostate cancer cells to proliferate. Some studies have also found that high levels of calcium (much more than typically consumed in the average diet) seem to increase the risk. Dr. Marc Garnick, editor in chief of the *Annual*, cautions his patients against taking more than 1,100 milligrams of calcium per day. (For references, see "Diet and prostate cancer risk," at left.)

As for alcohol and prostate cancer risk, studies have produced conflicting results. In 2018, researchers reported that men who had consumed at least seven alcoholic beverages a week between the ages of 15 and 49 had more than three times the risk of aggressive cancer than men who didn't drink at all. Yet a 2019 study showed that alcohol use was also associated with slightly *lower* odds of dying from prostate cancer, and that moderate intake of red wine specifically was associated with protection against cancer progression. However, a combined analysis of data from 83 published papers, performed by a different research group, detected slightly *higher* risks from drinking moderate amounts of red wine—and a protective effect from moderate white wine consumption. A 2020 analysis of studies in the published literature reached similar conclusions. Taken together, the evidence suggests that alcohol use in moderation poses little to no risk of prostate cancer. (For references, see "Alcohol and prostate cancer risk," at left.)

Smoking. Smoking isn't as strongly associated with prostate cancer as it is with cancers of the lung, kidney, and bladder. But results from a large analysis published in 2018 show that smokers do have a higher risk of worse outcomes from the disease. The investigators compiled data from six studies with a total of 22,549 men who had been followed for at least six years after treatment for localized prostate cancer. Compared with men who never smoked, the smokers had a 40% higher risk of biochemical recurrence after treatment and an 89% higher risk of death from prostate cancer. Former smokers who had quit within the prior six years had an elevated risk of relapse, but not of metastatic disease or death from prostate cancer. And men who had stopped smoking more than 10 years before a prostate cancer diagnosis had a risk profile similar to that of men who never smoked. (For reference, see "Smoking and prostate cancer risk," at left.)

Diet and prostate cancer risk

Allott EH, Arab L, Su LJ, et al. Saturated Fat Intake and Prostate Cancer Aggressiveness: Results from the Population-Based North Carolina–Louisiana Prostate Cancer Project. *Prostate Cancer and Prostatic Diseases* 2017;20(1):48–54. PMID: 27595916.

Fu BC, Tabung FK, Pernar CH, et al. Insulinemic and Inflammatory Dietary Patterns and Risk of Prostate Cancer. *European Urology* 2021;79(3):405–12. PMID: 33422354.

Labbé DP, Zadra G, Yang M, et al. High-Fat Diet Fuels Prostate Cancer Progression by Rewiring the Metabolome and Amplifying the MYC Program. *Nature Communications* 2019;10(1):4358. PMID: 31554818.

Murtola TJ, Kasurinen TVJ, Talala K, et al. Serum Cholesterol and Prostate Cancer Risk in the Finnish Randomized Study of Screening for Prostate Cancer. *Prostate Cancer and Prostatic Diseases* 2019;22(1)66–76. PMID: 30214034.

Pascual-Geler M, Urquiza-Salvat N, Cozar JM, et al. The Influence of Nutritional Factors on Prostate Cancer Incidence and Aggressiveness. *Aging Male* 2018;21(1):31–39. PMID: 28929838.

Alcohol and prostate cancer risk

Downer MK, Kenfield SA, Stampfer MJ, et al. Alcohol Intake and Risk of Lethal Prostate Cancer in the Health Professionals Follow-Up Study. *Journal of Clinical Oncology* 2019;37(17):1499–511. PMID: 31026211.

Hong S, Khil H, Lee, DH, et al. Alcohol Consumption and the Risk of Prostate Cancer: A Dose-Response Meta-Analysis. *Nutrients* 2020;12(8):2188. PMID: 32717903.

Michael J, Howard LE, Markt SC, et al. Early-Life Alcohol Intake and High-Grade Prostate Cancer: Results from an Equal-Access, Racially Diverse Biopsy Cohort. *Cancer Prevention Research* 2018;11(10):621–28. PMID: 30139875.

Vartolomei MD, Kimura S, Ferro M, et al. The Impact of Moderate Wine Consumption on the Risk of Developing Prostate Cancer. *Clinical Epidemiology* 2018;10:431–44. PMID: 29713200.

Smoking and prostate cancer risk

Foerster B, Pozo C, Abufaraj M, et al. Association of Smoking Status with Recurrence, Metastasis, and Mortality Among Patients with Localized Prostate Cancer Undergoing Prostatectomy or Radiotherapy: A Systematic Review and Meta-Analysis. *JAMA Oncology* 2018;4(7):953–61. PMID: 29800115.

PubMed See page 120.

Ejaculation frequency. In 2016, Harvard researchers published the strongest evidence yet that men who ejaculate frequently have a lower risk of prostate cancer. In a large, ongoing study, men ages 20 to 29 and those 40 to 49 who ejaculated more than 21 times per month had a 20% lower prostate cancer risk than those who ejaculated four to seven times a month. It's not clear why frequent ejaculation is protective, although some experts believe the release of semen flushes harmful substances from the prostate. A follow-up study by the same research team in 2018 supported that hypothesis: it showed that carcinogenic substances may accumulate in the prostate between ejaculations and alter the expression of genes within the gland's cells. (For references, see "Ejaculation and prostate cancer risk," page 42.)

Other factors. Researchers have examined other factors that might play a role in the development of prostate cancer—including sexually transmitted diseases, prostatitis, and vasectomy (for additional information, see "Do vasectomies raise the risk of prostate cancer?" at right)—but study findings have been inconsistent, and no firm conclusions have been drawn.

Can prostate cancer be prevented?

Knowing what increases a man's risk for prostate cancer is not the same as knowing how to prevent it. The biology of prostate cancer development is incredibly complex. Furthermore, any realistic advice about prevention has to be tailored to two different groups: men who want to reduce their risk of developing prostate cancer in the first place (primary prevention) and those who want to reduce the chances of a cancer recurrence (secondary prevention). This section discusses primary prevention of prostate cancer, with an emphasis on medications called 5-alpha-reductase inhibitors. For information about secondary prevention, see "Take charge of your condition," page 117.

5-alpha-reductase inhibitors

Many researchers and doctors hoped that finasteride (Proscar) and dutasteride (Avodart)—medications that are commonly used to treat benign prostatic hyperplasia (BPH)—would be the pharmaceutical wish-come-true for prostate cancer prevention. These drugs inhibit an enzyme called 5-alpha reductase type 2, which the body uses to convert testosterone into a more potent hormone, dihydrotestosterone (DHT). DHT not only promotes the growth of normal prostate tissue but also fuels the growth of tumors.

The FDA has warned since 2011 that finasteride and dutasteride might increase the risk of aggressive prostate cancer.

Follow-up research has generated conflicting results. An updated analysis published in 2019 with more than 18 years of follow-up found there were *fewer* prostate cancer deaths among men treated with finasteride than there were among men who took a placebo, despite the slightly higher rate of aggressive prostate cancer. Then a 2020 analysis found no evidence of either increased risk of diagnosis or death from prostate cancer. (For references, see "5-alpha-reductase inhibitors and prostate cancer prevention," page 42.)

Do vasectomies raise the risk of prostate cancer?

A vasectomy is a surgical procedure in which the tubes that carry sperm are cut and sealed. Some data have suggested that this procedure could increase the risk of prostate cancer, but the evidence is mixed. A 2017 investigation that reviewed 53 studies with a total of more than 2.5 million men could find no evidence linking the birth control procedure to high-grade or advanced prostate cancer. The authors of that study emphasized that worries over prostate cancer should not preclude men from getting a vasectomy.

More recently, a Danish study of more than two million men published in 2020 linked vasectomy to small increases in prostate cancer risk over time, which the authors said was similar in magnitude to the risk of breast cancer among women who use oral contraceptives. But many scientists say risks of prostate cancer from vasectomy have not been conclusively shown.

Sources: Bhindi B, Wallis CJD, Nayan M, et al. The Association Between Vasectomy and Prostate Cancer: A Systematic Review and Meta-Analysis. *JAMA Internal Medicine* 2017;177(9):1273–86. PMID: 28715534.

Husby A, Wohlfahrt J, Melbye M. Vasectomy and Prostate Cancer Risk: A 38-Year Nationwide Cohort Study. *Journal of the National Cancer Institute* 2020;112(1):71–77. PMID: 31119294.

Ejaculation and prostate cancer risk

Rider JR, Wilson KM, Sinnott JA, et al. Ejaculation Frequency and Risk of Prostate Cancer: Updated Results with an Additional Decade of Follow-Up. *European Urology* 2016;70(6):974–82. PMID: 27033442.

Sinnott JA, Brumberg K, Wilson KM, et al. Differential Gene Expression in Prostate Tissue According to Ejaculation Frequency. *European Urology* 2018;74(5):545–48. PMID: 29784192.

5-alpha-reductase inhibitors and prostate cancer prevention

Garnick MB. More on Long-Term Effects of Finasteride on Prostate Cancer Mortality. *New England Journal of Medicine* 2019;380(20):e38. PMID: 31091399.

Goodman PJ, Tangen CM, Darke AK, et al. Long-Term Effects of Finasteride on Prostate Cancer Mortality. *New England Journal of Medicine* 2019;380(4):393–94. PMID: 30673548.

Knijnk PG, Brum PW, Cachoeira ET, et al. The Impact of 5α-Reductase Inhibitors on Mortality in a Prostate Cancer Chemoprevention Setting: A Meta-Analysis. *World Journal of Urology* 2021;39(2):365–76. PMID: 32314009.

Sarkar RR, Parsons JK, Bryant AK, et al. Association of Treatment with 5α-Reductase Inhibitors with Time to Diagnosis and Mortality in Prostate Cancer. *JAMA Internal Medicine* 2019;179(6):812–19. PMID: 31058923.

Thompson IM Jr, Goodman PJ, Tangen CM, et al. Long-Term Survival of Participants in the Prostate Cancer Prevention Trial. *New England Journal of Medicine* 2013;369(7):603–10. PMID: 23944298.

Men who do take a 5-alpha-reductase inhibitor should be aware that these drugs lower PSA levels in blood by about 50%. If you get a PSA test while taking one of these drugs, your doctor should compensate for this effect of the drug by doubling your PSA measurement and using that figure to estimate whether further testing is needed. Evidence in support of this strategy was published in 2019. For that study, researchers looked at records for 80,875 men who had been diagnosed with prostate cancer between 2001 and 2015. They found that diagnoses were delayed by an average of 3.6 years in men taking one of these drugs for BPH, and that the delays often led to worse cancer outcomes. Anyone taking finasteride or dutasteride for BPH should talk about the pros and cons of those drugs with the prescribing physician, and PSA levels should be monitored closely. If PSA levels go up, remain level, or fail to decline by at least 50%, a biopsy may be in order.

Finasteride is also the active ingredient in Propecia, a drug used to treat baldness. Should that be a cause for concern among men taking Propecia? One of the studies on which the FDA based its warning tested a 5-mg dose of finasteride. However, a Propecia pill contains just 1 mg of the drug. It's not known whether finasteride in that amount will affect prostate cancer risk.

It's important to note that some men experience mood changes and persistent problems with sexual function after taking finasteride. The condition even has a name—post-finasteride syndrome (PFS)—and among its many reported symptoms are libido loss, erectile dysfunction, depression, panic attacks, and anxiety. A 2017 study found that 5-alpha-reductase inhibitors slightly increased the risk of depression, especially during the first 18 months of treatment. Yet the evidence is not conclusive: a 2019 review of studies enrolling a combined 209,940 men showed that the risk of depression from taking the medications was not significantly elevated, though the authors cautioned that definitive evidence would require a study that tracks patients' mental health going forward in time. Unfortunately, no one knows what could cause PFS, although new research in animals suggests the disorder might result from altered steroid levels in the brain, or perhaps from drug-induced changes to the gut's normal bacterial flora. (For references, see "Side effects of 5-alpha-reductase inhibitors," page 43.)

Other potential preventive agents

Other drugs and vitamins have been proposed as potential cancer-prevention agents, but there is not overwhelming evidence to support such claims. In fact, vitamin E supplementation actually increased the rate of prostate cancer development when it was tested in a rigorous fashion.

Vitamin D. Vitamin D can be obtained through sun exposure and by eating fatty fish and certain dairy products, such as fortified milk, as well as in supplements. A number of studies have correlated low vitamin D levels with various cancers, including higher risks of high-grade, more advanced prostate tumors. Sufficient intake of vitamin D might therefore be one potential way to reduce your overall risk, although the evidence is not conclusive and some studies have shown no prostate cancer prevention or treatment benefits from vitamin D supplements.

Statins. By reducing cholesterol (thereby reducing levels of testosterone, which requires cholesterol for its synthesis), statins may exert anti-cancer effects. A review article published in 2017 concluded that statins might lower prostate cancer risk by inhibiting tumor growth directly. Then in 2020, after scouring records from over 12,700 men who had been diagnosed with high-risk prostate cancer, scientists reported that statins given together with the diabetes drug metformin cut the risk of dying from any cause by a third. Metformin by itself had no similar effect. (For references, see "Possible agents to prevent prostate cancer," below right.) Still, according to Dr. Garnick, there is insufficient evidence to justify statin or metformin use for prostate cancer prevention at this time.

Diet

"What can I eat—and what foods should I avoid—to reduce my risk for prostate cancer?" This is one of the most common questions physicians hear from men concerned about prostate health. There is evidence that certain foods or dietary patterns may have protective effects, but it's suggestive, not definitive. (For references, see "Food and prostate cancer prevention," bottom right.)

Fruits and vegetables. Diets rich in fruits and vegetables may reduce the risk of prostate cancer. Carotenoids, compounds that occur naturally in certain plants, have antioxidant properties that may protect the body against unstable molecules that damage DNA. One frequently mentioned carotenoid is lycopene, the compound that gives tomatoes their bright red hue. Epidemiologic research has shown a correlation between eating tomato-based foods and lower prostate cancer risk. Pasta lovers will like this: two servings of tomato sauce a week seem to be enough to give some protection. But lycopene supplements have flopped in studies.

The Mediterranean diet. Prostate cancer death rates are much lower in the Mediterranean countries of southern Europe than in Scandinavia, Great Britain, and other parts of Europe. Any number of reasons could explain the difference, but the foods men eat might be one of them. The classic Mediterranean diet includes lots of fruits and vegetables, whole grains, and nuts, with olive oil instead of butter, and fish and poultry instead of red meat. Many studies show that eating that way limits chronic low-grade inflammation and contributes to good health, especially when it comes to preventing heart disease and stroke. And a 2021 investigation showed the Mediterranean diet may also protect against cancer progression among men with localized prostate cancer who choose to monitor their disease with active surveillance instead of having it treated right away; the study did not address primary prevention.

Fish. Large prospective studies have found that men who eat moderate to high amounts of fish were less likely to develop prostate cancer or die from it compared with men who do not eat fish. The protective benefits were thought to come from eating omega-3 fatty acids, which are naturally present in fish. But in 2017, Canadian researchers pulled together dozens of studies looking into possible links between prostate cancer and omega-3s, and concluded that the combined evidence was insufficient to draw a convincing connection.

Side effects of 5-alpha-reductase inhibitors

Basaria S, Jasuja R, Huang G, et al. Characteristics of Men Who Report Persistent Sexual Symptoms After Finasteride Use for Hair Loss. *Journal of Clinical Endocrinology & Metabolism* 2016;101(12):4669–80. PMID: 27662439.

Kiguradze T, Temps WH, Yarnold PR, et al. Persistent Erectile Dysfunction in Men Exposed to the 5α-Reductase Inhibitors, Finasteride, or Dutasteride. *PeerJ* 2017;5:e3020. PMID: 28289563.

Kim JH, Shim SR, Khandwala Y, et al. Risk of Depression After 5 Alpha Reductase Inhibitor Medication: Meta-Analysis. *World Journal of Men's Health* 2019;38(4):535–44. PMID: 31190484.

Welk B, McArthur E, Ordon M, et al. Association of Suicidality and Depression with 5α-Reductase Inhibitors. *JAMA Internal Medicine* 2017;177(5):683–91. PMID: 28319231.

Possible agents to prevent prostate cancer

Alfaqih MA, Allott EH, Hamilton RJ, et al. The Current Evidence on Statin Use and Prostate Cancer Prevention: Are We There Yet? *Nature Reviews Urology* 2017;14(2):107–19. PMID: 27779230.

Tan XL, E JU, Rebbeck TR, et al. Individual and Joint Effects of Metformin and Statins on Mortality Among Patients with High-Risk Prostate Cancer. *Cancer Medicine* 2020;9(7):2379–89. PMID: 32035002.

Food and prostate cancer prevention

Aucoin M, Cooley K, Knee C, et al. Fish-Derived Omega-3 Fatty Acids and Prostate Cancer: A Systematic Review. *Integrative Cancer Therapies* 2017;16(1):32–62. PMID: 27365385.

Gregg JR, Zhang X, Chapin BF, et al. Adherence to the Mediterranean Diet and Grade Group Progression in Localized Prostate Cancer: An Active Surveillance Cohort. *Cancer* 2021;127(5):720–28. PMID: 33411364.

Kenfield SA, DuPre N, Richman EL, et al. Mediterranean Diet and Prostate Cancer Risk and Mortality in the Health Professionals Follow-Up Study. *European Urology* 2014;65(5):887–94. PMID: 23962747.

PubMed See page 120.

Exercise and prostate cancer prevention

Pernar CH, Ebot EM, Pettersson A, et al. A Prospective Study of the Association Between Physical Activity and Risk of Prostate Cancer Defined by Clinical Features and TMPRSS2:ERG. *European Urology* 2019;76(1):33–40. PMID: 30301696.

Plym A, Zhang Y, Stopsack K, et al. Can the Genetic Risk of Prostate Cancer Be Attenuated by a Healthy Lifestyle? Presented at the 2021 American Association for Cancer Research Annual Meeting (Virtual). Abstract No. 822.

Exercise

Some evidence suggests that men can lower their likelihood of getting prostate cancer with regular exercise. In 2019, Harvard scientists published findings on 49,160 men who were followed in a national study from 1986 until 2012. The men answered questions twice a year about their diet, health, and physical activity. A total of 6,411 of the participants developed prostate cancer, and 888 developed an aggressive form of the disease. The study showed that men who engaged most frequently in vigorous activity had a 30% lower risk of developing advanced prostate cancer and a 25% lower risk of dying from prostate cancer compared with men who exercised the least. The reduction also carried over to men who tested positive for a gene fusion called TMPRSS2:ERG that is associated with higher risk of prostate cancer, showing that exercise can be protective even for men who may be genetically prone to developing the disease.

According to another Harvard study, reported in 2021, sticking to a healthy lifestyle—maintaining an optimal weight, engaging in vigorous physical activity, not smoking, limiting the intake of processed meats such as bacon and hot dogs, and eating lots of tomatoes and fatty fish—cut the risk of lethal prostate cancer even among men who are at high genetic risk for the disease. (For references, see "Exercise and prostate cancer prevention," above left.)

Symptoms of prostate cancer

Many men with prostate cancer have no symptoms. But because the prostate gland is enlarged both in cancer and in nonmalignant conditions such as BPH, these very different conditions share many of the same symptoms. Contact your physician if you notice any of the following signs or symptoms:

- a need to urinate frequently, particularly at night
- difficulty starting or stopping urination
- a weak or interrupted urinary stream
- an inability to urinate
- pain or burning when you urinate
- painful ejaculation
- blood in your urine or ejaculate
- frequent pain or stiffness in your lower back, hips, or upper thighs.

Screening

There are two types of screening for prostate cancer. The first one—the digital rectal exam—is well accepted among doctors. The second one is common, but controversial.

Digital rectal examination

In case you had any doubt, the word "digital" in digital rectal exam (DRE) doesn't have anything to do with computers or data. Rather, the digit in the digital rectal exam is the doctor's lubricated, gloved finger inserted into the rectum. Because the prostate sits in front of the rectum, the doctor can feel part of it through the rectal wall. A normal prostate is small—about an inch and a half from side to side—and feels smooth and rubbery. Swelling, lumps, firm knots, or abnormally textured areas may indicate prostate cancer or another condition.

Early cancerous tumors are often too small to detect during a DRE, and some are located in areas a doctor's finger can't reach. Only the back of the gland can be felt, but this is where most prostate cancers develop. For these reasons, clinicians who use DRE alone to screen for prostate cancer may miss the smallest and most treatable tumors. At the same time, small tumors that can't be felt by the physician may be less likely to cause future problems.

Prostate-specific antigen (PSA) test

Most men with prostate cancer don't have any symptoms in the initial stages of the disease (see "Symptoms of prostate cancer," at left). And, as noted, the DRE doesn't find small cancers or those in the front (anterior) portion of the gland. So when the PSA test was introduced as a screening test during the 1990s, it took off. The idea of catching cancer early, when it's more treatable, is a powerful one, and studies show that PSA tests save roughly one life for every 1,000 men screened over 10 years.

But the PSA test has proved to be problematic, because PSA is not solely produced by cancer cells. Normal prostate cells produce it, too, and there's always a small amount of PSA circulating in the blood. When the prostate is irritated or damaged or has turned cancerous, more PSA leaks into the bloodstream. As a result, elevated PSA levels can accompany the noncancerous conditions BPH and prostatitis, or a number of other factors such as recent sexual activity, bike riding, recent urinary infections, or recent urinary catheterization (see "What causes PSA levels to rise or fall?" on page 46). And some men's prostates naturally release more of the protein into the blood. So PSA is true to its name; it's specific to the prostate, but not to cancer.

That means a high PSA level can cause a false alarm—the medical term is a false positive. But the opposite problem also exists. The PSA test misses cancer about 15% of the time—the medical term is a false negative. To help get a sense of what's normal for a particular patient, some experts argue that men should at least get a baseline PSA measurement during their 40s or early 50s and then have more tests later, depending on the initial results and other risk factors. Either way, men should be aware of the potential risks and benefits of PSA screening before making such a decision.

Even if the PSA test performs as desired and leads to further tests that confirm prostate cancer, that cancer may be very slow-growing (indolent), so that it wouldn't have caused any harm. Doctors use the term "overdiagnosis" to refer to detection of a prostate cancer that wouldn't have caused any problems and would have gone undetected were it not for screening. By some calculations, 23% to 57% of screen-detected prostate cancers fall into the overdiagnosis category, and the figures are highest for older men.

If overdiagnosis merely failed to deliver benefits, that would be one thing. But it can also lead to harm. If a man has an elevated PSA level, doctors often order a prostate biopsy, which can cause pain, bleeding, or other complications—the most worrisome being infection, which can be serious enough to require hospitalization. (For more information on biopsies, see "The biopsy procedure," page 52.) Furthermore, once diagnosed, many men choose to undergo treatment—prompting worries that an excessive number of them are being treated for prostate cancer that may never be life-threatening and are risking serious treatment-related complications.

Accordingly, in 2012, the USPSTF issued guidelines recommending against routine PSA screening, regardless of age, race, or family history. Initially, cancer cases fell, presumably because many cases weren't being detected. But studies have since found that new diagnoses of advanced prostate cancer rose after that recommendation. (For references, see "PSA screening and diagnosis rates," at right.)

The USPSTF softened its anti-testing stance in 2018, largely because men with low-risk prostate cancers flagged by PSA screening are increasingly opting for active surveillance rather than immediate treatment, thereby avoiding unnecessary cancer therapies and their associated harms, perhaps indefinitely. However, the true long-term effects of reduced PSA screening will not be known for years—and according to Dr. Garnick, they may never be known.

PSA screening and diagnosis rates

Bell N, Gorber SC, Shane A, et al. Recommendations on Screening for Prostate Cancer with the Prostate-Specific Antigen Test. *Canadian Medical Association Journal* 2014;186(16):1225–34. PMID: 25349003.

Borza T, Kaufman SR, Shahinian VB, et al. Sharp Decline in Prostate Cancer Treatment Among Men in the General Population, but Not Among Diagnosed Men. *Health Affairs (Millwood)* 2017;36(1):108–15. PMID: 28069853.

Butler SS, Muralidhar V, Zhao SG, et al. Prostate Cancer Incidence Across Stage, NCCN Risk Groups, and Age Before and After USPSTF Grade D Recommendations Against Prostate-Specific Antigen Screening in 2012. *Cancer* 2020;126(4):717–24. PMID: 31794057.

Carter HB, Albertsen PC, Barry MJ, et al. Early Detection of Prostate Cancer: AUA Guideline. *Journal of Urology* 2013;190(2):419–26. PMID: 23659877.

Magnani CJ, Li K, Seto T, et al. PSA Testing Use and Prostate Cancer Diagnostic Stage After the 2012 U.S. Preventive Services Task Force Guideline Changes. *Journal of the National Comprehensive Cancer Network* 2019;17(7):795–803. PMID: 31319390.

Qaseem A, Barry MJ, Demberg TD, et al. Screening for Prostate Cancer: A Guidance Statement from the Clinical Guidelines Committee of the American College of Physicians. *Annals of Internal Medicine* 2013;158(10):761–69. PMID: 23567643.

U.S. Preventive Services Task Force, Grossman DC, Curry SJ, et al. Screening for Prostate Cancer: US Preventive Services Task Force Recommendation Statement. *JAMA* 2018;319(18):1901–13. PMID: 29801017.

Wolf AM, Wender RC, Etzioni RB, et al. American Cancer Society Guideline for the Early Detection of Prostate Cancer: Update 2010. *CA: A Cancer Journal for Clinicians* 2010;60(2):70–98. PMID: 20200110.

Zavaski ME, Meyer CP, Sammon JD, et al. Differences in Prostate-Specific Antigen Testing Among Urologists and Primary Care Physicians Following the 2012 USPSTF Recommendations. *JAMA Internal Medicine* 2016;176(4):546–47. PMID: 26857148.

PubMed See page 120.

As in most controversies, the truth may lie somewhere in the middle, as reflected by growing consensus around the issue of screening:

- The American College of Physicians, the national organization for internists, recommends that doctors inform men ages 50 to 69 about what it describes as the "limited potential benefits and substantial harms" of screening.
- The USPSTF's revised guidelines, issued in 2018, recommend that clinicians inform men ages 55 to 69 about the potential risks and benefits of PSA screening. They advise against screening men over 70 and give no recommendation for men younger than 55.
- The American Urological Association (AUA) guidelines advise against routine screening and recommend "shared decision-making" (a process by which the patient and doctor work together to reach an agreement on how to proceed) only for men ages 55 to 69.
- The ACS recommends against screening until men discuss the associated uncertainties with their doctors. The ACS position is that these discussions should begin at age 50 for men at average risk, at age 45 for men at higher risk (such as African Americans or men with a father, son, or brother who was diagnosed with prostate cancer), and at age 40 for men who have more than one first-degree relative with prostate cancer.
- The Canadian Task Force on Preventive Health Care strongly recommends against PSA screening among men younger than 55 or older than 70, and they make a

What causes PSA levels to rise or fall?

These factors typically produce a substantial or sustained rise in PSA:

- benign prostatic hyperplasia (BPH)
- prostatitis
- urinary tract infections
- prostate biopsies
- prostate cancer.

These factors sometimes produce a small or temporary rise in PSA:

- ejaculation
- a digital rectal examination (DRE)
- a urinary catheter and bladder examination
- vigorous bike riding
- warm climates
- changes in laboratories or testing methods
- hepatitis
- bypass surgery.

These factors typically produce a substantial or sustained decrease in PSA:

- therapy with finasteride (Proscar) or dutasteride (Avodart)
- use of finasteride in a smaller-dose formulation (Propecia) as a treatment for hair loss
- prostate cancer surgery.

These factors sometimes produce a small or temporary decrease in PSA:

- therapy with a statin drug (for cholesterol) or a thiazide diuretic (for blood pressure)
- therapy with a nonsteroidal anti-inflammatory drug (NSAID)
- obesity
- changes in laboratories or testing methods.

weaker recommendation against it for men ages 55 to 70. Moreover, they urge doctors not to discuss PSA screening with men younger than 55 or older than 70, unless a man raises the topic first. Men ages 55 to 70 may choose to be screened, the Canadian guidelines state, if they place a higher value on the small potential in reduction of death than on the higher risk of potential harms that come with screening.

Should you be tested?

It's important to recognize that controversies over the PSA test focus solely on routine screening for potential cancer—not on the use of the PSA test to gauge whether a particular prostate cancer treatment is working. Both surgery and hormonal therapy should lower PSA levels substantially. (So should radiation, but to a lesser extent.) If levels rise after treatment, it could mean these interventions haven't been successful. PSA testing therefore plays an important role during treatment for prostate cancer.

The question is whether or not to use the PSA test to screen for prostate cancer in the first place. Here are some factors to consider: Since Black men are at higher risk of developing and dying from prostate cancer than men of other races, they might therefore consider screening at younger ages. Similarly, men who have first-degree relatives with the disease might consider early screening, especially if they also have genetic risk factors for prostate cancer. (For reference, see "Early screening," page 48.) However, there are no good data yet showing that earlier screening is beneficial in these populations.

While a combination of PSA testing and DRE may nearly double the detection rate for early-stage prostate cancer, low-grade, low-volume cancers may progress so slowly that they pose no immediate threat, especially to older men who may die of other causes long before the prostate cancer would have progressed. So, an elevated PSA level may cause needless worry and treatment.

Some PSA test advocates point out that the test not only finds many more prostate cancers in early stages than was possible in the past, but also that the death rate from the disease in the United States began to drop not long after the PSA test became a routine part of a medical exam in most men over age 50. Others, however, attribute the decline to factors such as better treatments and changes in the American diet.

Finally, in many cases, a suspicious PSA test will lead to additional procedures (such as ultrasound, MRI, and biopsies) to determine if cancer is present, and possibly to surgery or radiation. Some men—particularly older men with slow-growing prostate cancer—may be treated needlessly and suffer from complications of treatment, such as impotence and incontinence.

That's why, before you choose to have the test, it's extremely important for you to understand the uncertainties and decisions you will face (see "Take-home messages about PSA screening," at right). And if you decide to have a PSA test, keep in mind that PSA levels can vary for reasons unrelated to cancer. Before acting on a surprisingly high PSA, consider repeating the test in a month or two to confirm the result.

What constitutes a high PSA reading? Most experts agree that a PSA level is abnormal once it rises above 4 nanograms per milliliter (ng/ml) of blood. Studies have

Take-home messages about PSA screening

- Screening doesn't lower your risk of having prostate cancer; it increases the chance you'll find out if you have it.
- PSA testing can detect localized or microscopic cancers that a digital rectal examination (DRE) would miss.
- A "normal" PSA level of 4 ng/ml or below doesn't guarantee that you are cancer-free; in about 15% of men with a PSA below 4 ng/ml, a biopsy will reveal prostate cancer.
- An elevated PSA level may prompt you to seek further diagnostic tests and, if cancer is found, lead to treatment, resulting in possible urinary and sexual side effects.
- Conditions other than cancer—BPH and prostatitis, for example—can elevate your PSA level.
- PSA levels can increase after ejaculation or other activities that stimulate or jostle the prostate, such as bike riding, horseback riding, or riding an all-terrain vehicle. Men who choose to get a PSA test should abstain from such activities for three days prior to getting tested.
- PSA levels are generally lower in obese men than they are in lean men.
- Levels of free PSA—meaning PSA that is not bound to proteins in blood—tend to fall in men who have prostate cancer as opposed to more benign conditions. A separate test of free PSA is most helpful when the regular PSA test level is between 4 and 10 ng/ml.

suggested that a man who has a PSA of 4 to 10 ng/ml has a 25% chance of having prostate cancer; if his PSA is greater than 10, the likelihood increases to more than 50%. But some studies suggest that the traditional cutoff point of 4 ng/ml may be too high. So we should probably think of PSA values as being on a continuum, with higher values associated with a greater likelihood of having prostate cancer.

Variations on the PSA test

Rather than subject everyone with an elevated PSA reading to a biopsy, some doctors do additional tests that involve more detailed interpretations of PSA levels.

Free PSA. PSA circulates in the blood in two forms—either bound to other proteins or unbound (free). Several studies suggest that men with elevated PSA levels who have a very low percentage of free PSA are more likely to have prostate cancer than a benign prostate condition. By contrast, higher circulating levels of free PSA are typically associated with benign prostate conditions. The free PSA level doesn't give a definitive answer, but it may be useful when considering whether a biopsy is the appropriate next step. Many doctors recommend biopsies in men with a free PSA level of 10% or less and advise men to consider a biopsy if the free PSA level is between 10% and 25%.

PSA velocity. Some physicians rely on measures known as serial PSA or PSA velocity, which track how much the PSA reading increases from one test to the next. Physicians must obtain at least four values over time, starting with a baseline measurement and then additional measures taken at six, 12, and then 18 to 24 months. PSA scores tend to rise more rapidly in men with cancer than in those with BPH, and some research has shown that men with prostate cancer who have rapid increases in PSA are more likely to die from the disease than those with slower-rising levels. (For references, see "PSA velocity," at left.) However, PSA velocity is controversial, and evidence shows it can lead to large numbers of unnecessary biopsies. According to Dr. Garnick, PSA velocity adds little to the individual PSA value.

Prostate Health Index. In 2012, the FDA approved the Prostate Health Index (PHI) for use in men 50 and older with PSA levels between 4 and 10 ng/ml whose rectal exams do not show evidence of cancer. About 25% of men with PSA levels in this range have cancer; the other 75% do not. The PHI combines three different measurements: total PSA, free PSA, and a type of PSA called proPSA that has a different number of amino acids. Developers of the proPSA test claim that this type of PSA is highly specific to prostate cancer. The measurements are incorporated into a formula that generates the combined index.

Research suggests that the PHI may have greater specificity—that is, an ability to predict who does not have prostate cancer—than traditional PSA measures. A 2017 study of 345 men screened at Johns Hopkins University Hospital found that the PHI was a better predictor of prostate cancer than PSA by itself, and that rising PHI scores also predicted more aggressive cancer. The authors suggested that incorporating the PHI into cancer screening could reduce unnecessary biopsies, without sacrificing the detection of high-grade cancers. A study with 1,189 men published the following year bolsters this view—biopsy procedures were significantly reduced among men with

Early screening

Xu X, Kharazmi E, Tian Y, et al. Risk of Prostate Cancer in Relatives of Prostate Cancer Patients in Sweden: A Nationwide Cohort Study. *PLOS Medicine* 2021;18(6):e2003616. PMID: 34061847.

PSA velocity

Vickers AJ, Thompson IM, Klein E, et al. A Commentary on PSA Velocity and Doubling Time for Clinical Decisions in Prostate Cancer. *Urology* 2014;83(3):592–98. PMID: 24581521.

Vickers AJ, Till C, Tangen CM, et al. An Empirical Evaluation of Guidelines on Prostate-Specific Antigen Velocity in Prostate Cancer Detection. *Journal of the National Cancer Institute* 2011;103(6):462–69. PMID: 21350221.

Wallner LP, Frencher SK, Hsu JW, et al. Changes in Serum Prostate-Specific Antigen Levels and the Identification of Prostate Cancer in a Large Managed Care Population. *BJU International* 2013;111(8):1245–52. PMID: 23320750.

PSA levels in the range of 4 to 10 ng/ml and nonsuspicious DRE findings (not indicative of cancer) who also had a PHI test.

The PHI test is also being used to check for tumor growth among men on active surveillance, which is an alternative to immediate treatment for low-risk prostate cancer. A study with 253 men on active surveillance, published in 2020, showed that PHI combined with multiparametric magnetic resonance imaging (see "Special MRI imaging techniques," page 50) detected growing cancers nearly as accurately as prostate biopsies. The evidence suggests that the two tests given together can reduce biopsy frequency for men on active surveillance. Still, the PHI has not been widely adopted, and Dr. Garnick urges caution with this test until more data become available to validate it. (For references, see "Prostate Health Index," at right.)

4Kscore. The 4Kscore is similar to the PHI. The PSA protein is a member of a family of enzymes called kallikreins. Like the PHI, the 4Kscore combines three different measurements of PSA but adds a fourth factor, a fellow kallikrein called human kallikrein 2. So, the name 4Kscore comes from the fact that four kallikrein measurements are included in the formula. Several studies have shown that the 4Kscore correlates with the biopsy outcome and therefore might help men decide whether to proceed with a biopsy or choose active surveillance. (For references, see "4Kscore," below right.)

Imaging

Many prostate cancers today are diagnosed at the earliest stages, when a tumor may be no bigger than a pea. Radiologists are continually trying to improve the imaging techniques that enable physicians to better understand how extensive a prostate cancer is and where it is located in the gland—details that can be used along with other clinical information, such as the biopsy findings that confirm a cancer diagnosis, to help predict how aggressive a tumor is.

Ultrasound

In conventional ultrasound procedures, a probe placed against the skin sends painless, ultra-high-frequency sound waves into the body. As the waves strike internal organs, they produce echo patterns that a computer converts into images (sonograms) on a video screen. Transrectal ultrasonography (TRUS) is a way of creating an image of the prostate gland, using a probe, or ultrasound transducer, inserted into the rectum. Sound waves scan the prostate gland in two planes. The resulting pictures often serve as a guide for a biopsy of the prostate, helping to delineate the gland's anatomy and pinpoint any suspicious areas. Doctors may also use TRUS when they suspect prostate cancer based on an abnormal DRE or an elevated PSA.

Magnetic resonance imaging (MRI)

An MRI machine uses a very large magnet, a radio-wave transmitter, and a computer to construct detailed pictures of structures inside the body. Cancerous tissue has a different set of magnetic properties than normal tissue, and MRI can capture these differences.

Prostate Health Index

Ferro M, De Cobelli O, Lucarelli, et al. Beyond PSA: The Role of the Prostate Health Index. *International Journal of Molecular Science* 2020;21(4):1184. PMID: 32053990.

Loeb S, Catalona WJ. The Prostate Health Index: A New Test for the Detection of Prostate Cancer. *Therapeutic Advances in Urology* 2014;6(2):74–77. PMID: 24688603.

Schwen ZR, Mamawala M, Tosoian JJ, et al. Prostate Health Index and Multiparametric Magnetic Resonance Imaging to Predict Prostate Cancer Grade Reclassification in Active Surveillance. *British Journal of Urology* 2020;126(3):373–78. PMID: 32367635.

Tosoian JJ, Druskin SC, Andreas D, et al. Use of the Prostate Health Index for Detection of Prostate Cancer: Results from a Large Academic Practice. *Prostate Cancer and Prostatic Diseases* 2017;20(2):228–33. PMID: 28117387.

White J, Shenoy BV, Tutrone RF, et al. Clinical Utility of the Prostate Health Index (PHI) for Biopsy Decision Management in a Large Group Urology Practice Setting. *Prostate Cancer and Prostatic Diseases* 2018;21(1):78–84. PMID: 29158509.

4Kscore

Russo GI, Regis F, Castelli T, et al. A Systematic Review and Meta-Analysis of the Diagnostic Accuracy of Prostate Health Index and 4-Kallikrein Panel Score in Predicting Overall and High-Grade Prostate Cancer. *Clinical Genitourinary Cancer* 2017;15(4):429–39. PMID: 28111174.

Sjoberg DD, Vickers AJ, Assel M, et al. Twenty-Year Risk of Prostate Cancer Death by Midlife Prostate-Specific Antigen and a Panel of Four Kallikrein Markers in a Large Population-Based Cohort of Healthy Men. *European Urology* 2018;73(6):941–48. PMID: 29519548.

PubMed See page 120.

Imaging advances

Ahmed HU, El-Shater Bosaily A, Brown LC, et al. Diagnostic Accuracy of Multi-Parametric MRI and TRUS Biopsy in Prostate Cancer (PROMIS): A Paired Validating Confirmatory Study. *Lancet* 2017;389(10071):815–22. PMID: 28110982.

Bjurlin MA, Carroll PR, Eggener S, et al. Update of the Standard Operating Procedure on the Use of Multiparametric Magnetic Resonance Imaging for the Diagnosis, Staging, and Management of Prostate Cancer. *Journal of Urology* 2020;203(4):706–12. PMID: 31642740.

Branger N, Maubon T, Traumann M, et al. Is Negative Multiparametric Magnetic Resonance Imaging Really Able to Exclude Significant Prostate Cancer? The Real-Life Experience. *BJU International* 2017;119(3):449–55. PMID: 27618134.

Eldred-Evans D, Burak P, Connor MJ, et al. Population-Based Cancer Screening with Magnetic Resonance Imaging or Ultrasonography: The IP1-PROSTAGRAM Study. *JAMA Oncology* 2021;7(3):395–402. PMID: 33570542.

Lee SI, O'Shea A. Community-Based Screening for Prostate Cancer. A Role for Magnetic Resonance Imaging? *JAMA Oncology* 2021;7(3):402–3. PMID: 33570559.

Oppenheimer DC, Weinberg EP, Hollenberg GM, et al. Multiparametric Magnetic Resonance Imaging of Recurrent Prostate Cancer. *Journal of Clinical Imaging Science* 2016;6:18. PMID: 27195184.

Patel P, Want S, Siddiqui MM. The Use of Multiparametric Resonance Imaging (mpMRI) in the Detection, Evaluation, and Surveillance of Clinically Significant Prostate Cancer (csPCa). *Current Urology Reports* 2019;20(10):60. PMID: 31478113.

Stabile A, Giganti F, Rosenkrantz AB, et al. Multiparametric MRI for Prostate Cancer Diagnosis: Current Status and Future Directions. *Nature Reviews Urology* 2020;17(1):41–61. PMID: 31316185.

MRI of the prostate can be done with or without an endorectal coil, a thin wire covered with a small inflated balloon that's inserted in the rectum. Once the MRI machine is turned on, the coil receives the magnetic waves. The closer the coil is to the target tissue, the stronger the signal and the clearer the images. The endorectal coil can be uncomfortable, so the doctor may inject a muscle relaxant to help muscles in the rectal wall relax. Some patients also receive a mild sedative to ease any anxiety.

This imaging exam is not used for routine screening, but it can be helpful in certain situations. For example, if the PSA continues to rise but a biopsy doesn't detect cancer, MRI may pinpoint a suspicious area for a more targeted biopsy.

One of the reasons MRI is valuable is that it provides high-resolution images of the entire prostate gland—especially important when there is a question of how extensive a cancer is or whether it has spread. In 80% to 85% of men diagnosed with prostate cancer, the tumor is multifocal, meaning the cancer is in more than one location. MRI's ability to show the entire prostate, particularly the parts a clinician can't reach with a DRE, helps physicians determine how far the cancer has grown.

Special MRI imaging techniques. To improve the quality of the image, radiologists may inject a contrast agent, such as a dye, through an intravenous line. The contrast agent travels through the bloodstream and is absorbed by the prostate. Cancerous tissue absorbs the agent in a different way from other tissue, so the malignant tissue appears brighter on the scan than benign tissue.

Multiparametric MRI (MP-MRI) is a hybrid approach that combines several different MRI strategies and improves diagnostic accuracy compared with any individual MRI technique used alone. Using images from these scans, a skilled urologist can target a biopsy in an area that appears abnormal. Evidence is increasing that MP-MRI scanning may allow men on active surveillance for low-risk cancer to forgo repeat biopsies. During a 2017 study, 576 men with high PSA levels underwent MP-MRI of the prostate, followed by standard ultrasound-guided biopsy and a more invasive type of biopsy that samples the entire gland at 5-millimeter intervals. MP-MRI correctly identified prostate tumors in men who actually did have prostate cancer at least 89% of time and didn't miss a single intermediate- to high-risk tumor. If MP-MRI had been used to make decisions on whether or not to do a biopsy, 158 of the men (27%) would have avoided a diagnostic biopsy altogether. Indeed, guidelines issued by the European Association of Urology state that men with elevated PSA levels can skip diagnostic biopsies if their MP-MRI scans are normal, but only after discussing the pros and cons with a doctor. (Importantly, MP-MRI is an expensive and lengthy procedure that can require up to an hour to perform. It is generally available only in academic teaching hospitals, but will likely to increase in availability in the coming years. Equally important is the need to have a qualified radiologist who can read and interpret MP-MRI screening results.)

MRI spectroscopy analyzes the chemical composition of tissue. This technique provides metabolic information that can help distinguish between prostate cancer and benign prostatic tissue. At this point, MRI spectroscopy is used only at research centers. The equipment and the analytics needed preclude broader use. (For references, see "Imaging advances," above left.)

Positron emission tomography (PET)

PET scans typically measure the amount of blood sugar, or glucose, cells use. They are useful for identifying many types of cancers, but for reasons that aren't clear, prostate cancer cells don't use as much glucose as other types of cancer cells, so they don't stand out on PET scans as clearly. To solve this problem, researchers have been looking for tracer compounds that will preferentially attach to prostate cancer cells.

One FDA-approved imaging agent, known as choline C11, accumulates in prostate cancer cells that are metastasizing (spreading) in the body. A patient gets an injection of choline C11 shortly before a PET scan. As the cancer cells metabolize glucose, the choline C11 that has collected in them breaks down, producing beta decay, a type of radioactive energy that shows up clearly on PET scans. PET scans using choline C11 are approved for use in men whose PSA levels start to rise after surgery or radiation for prostate cancer. Called biochemical recurrence, this signifies that some cancer remains after treatment and may be spreading to the bones or lymph nodes, though it cannot be detected with conventional imaging.

In 2016, the FDA approved another radioactive PET scan tracer, called fluciclovine F18 (Axumin), also for use in men whose PSA levels rise after prostate cancer treatment.

Researchers have also reported promising results with newer radioactive tracers, including one called gallium-68 PSMA-11 that received FDA approval in 2020. This tracer binds to a protein called prostate-specific membrane antigen (PSMA) in the prostate cancer cell membrane. In 2019, researchers evaluated the tracer in a study with 635 men who had rising PSA levels after prostate cancer surgery. Results showed it could detect metastatic tumors with 84% accuracy. A 2020 review of 37 studies supported those results, as did findings from a clinical trial with 300 men who were given either the gallium PSMA scan or a conventional CT scan before surgical or radiation treatment for high-risk prostate cancer. The gallium PSMA scan in this case detected metastases with 92% accuracy, compared with the 65% accuracy achieved with the conventional method.

As of 2021, gallium PET scanning was available at only two academic hospitals in California. However, the FDA approved a second PSMA-binding PET tracer in 2021. Called piflufolastat F18 (Pylarify), it was approved for use in detecting metastatic or recurring prostate cancer, and is expected to be broadly available throughout the United States by early 2022. (For references, see "PET scan advances," above right.)

PSMA scans are particularly useful for diagnosing oligometastatic prostate cancer, which is defined by the presence of five or fewer metastases in the body that may not yet be visible with conventional imaging. Men who have this condition can be treated with new and highly targeted forms of radiation that treat tiny cancerous deposits and spare healthy surrounding tissues. (For more on this topic, see the Roundtable discussion, page 90.)

Biopsies and diagnosis

If your doctor suspects you have prostate cancer on the basis of an elevated PSA level or abnormal DRE, the next step in diagnosis is to have a biopsy. This procedure entails

PET scan advances

Durack JC, Alva AS, Preston MA, et al. A Prospective Phase II/III Study of PSMA-Targeted 18F-DCFPyL-PET/CT in Patients (pts) With Prostate Cancer (PCa) (OSPREY): A Subanalysis of Disease Staging Changes in PCa pts With Recurrence or Metastases on Conventional Imaging. Presented at the American Society of Clinical Oncology 2021 Genitourinary Cancers Symposium. Abstract No. 32.

Fendler WP, Calais J, Eiber M, et al. Assessment of 68Ga-PSMA-11 PET Accuracy in Localizing Recurrent Prostate Cancer: A Prospective Single-Arm Clinical Trial. *JAMA Oncology* 2019;5(6):856–63. PMID: 30920593.

Hofman MS, Lawrentschuk N, Francis RJ, et al. Prostate-Specific Membrane Antigen PET-CT in Patients with High Risk Prostate Cancer Before Curative-Intent Surgery or Radiotherapy (proPSMA): A Prospective, Randomized Multi-Center Study. *Lancet* 2020;395(10231):1208–16. PMID: 32209449.

Perera M, Papa N, Roberts M, et al. Gallium-68 Prostate-Specific Membrane Antigen Positron Emission Tomography in Advanced Prostate Cancer—Updated Diagnostic Utility, Sensitivity, Specificity, and Distribution of Prostate-Specific Membrane Antigen-avid Lesions: A Systematic Review and Meta-Analysis. *European Urology* 2020;77(4):403–17. PMID: 30773328.

PubMed See page 120.

removing small pieces of tissue from the prostate and sending them to a laboratory to check for cancerous cells. If cancer is found, the characteristics of the biopsied cells, along with findings from other tests, enable the doctor to classify its severity.

The biopsy procedure

Doctors may choose among several approaches for taking prostate biopsies, depending on such factors as the purpose of the biopsy, the location of the suspicious area, and the patient's health. (For references on the various procedures, see "Biopsy research," at left.)

Transrectal biopsy. The most common biopsy procedure is the transrectal ultrasound-guided (TRUS) biopsy. While you lie on your side, the doctor inserts an ultrasound probe into your rectum and scans the prostate. A separate spring-loaded device rapidly inserts a needle through the rectal wall into the prostate and retrieves a tiny tissue sample. The doctor uses the ultrasound image as a guide in taking biopsies from specific areas. The standard used to be six samples, or cores; that's why it was called the sextant biopsy. Now 10 to 12 cores are often taken. Some medical centers perform "saturation" biopsies that involve retrieving 20 to 30 samples, but the optimal number of cores remains uncertain.

After the ultrasound probe is introduced and before the biopsies are taken, the doctor may inject an anesthetic into the prostate, guided again by the ultrasound image. Even with anesthesia, you may feel a slight pinch when each tissue sample is taken. The procedure itself usually takes less than 15 minutes.

Transrectal biopsies have become standard practice for a reason. They can be done in an outpatient setting without general anesthesia. They're quick, relatively inexpensive, and safe the vast majority of the time. But they also have some drawbacks and risks. For example, 10% to 70% of men (yes, such a wide range indicates uncertainty) have blood in their semen (hematospermia) for about four to eight weeks after undergoing a standard TRUS biopsy. Hematospermia is a troubling—though usually harmless—side effect of this procedure. To avoid excessive bleeding, men are instructed not to take aspirin or similar drugs, such as ibuprofen (Advil, Motrin) and naproxen (Aleve), for a week before the biopsy. Up to 25% of men experience lower urinary tract symptoms (having to urinate often, poor stream, dribbling, and so on), although this is almost always a temporary problem. Repeat biopsies can also increase the likelihood of erectile dysfunction, especially in older men. (For references, see "Biopsy complications," page 53.)

TRUS biopsies can also have more serious consequences, particularly if fecal bacteria from the rectum are introduced into the prostate gland. The needle to collect the specimen goes through the rectum, so there's a chance that bacteria in the rectum will escape and spread to the bloodstream (septicemia). Indeed, post-biopsy infections are a growing problem. For a study published in 2018, researchers investigated complication rates in 26,254 men who had undergone a TRUS biopsy. About 2% of the men—530 in all—developed infections requiring hospitalization. These sorts of biopsies also come with a risk of urinary tract infections, especially for men who have had them before.

Biopsy research

Ahdoot M, Wilbur AR, Reese SE, et al. MRI-Targeted, Systematic, and Combined Biopsy for Prostate Cancer Diagnosis. *New England Journal of Medicine* 2020;382:917–28. PMID: 32130814.

Bjurlin MA, Carroll PR, Eggener S, et al. Update of the Standard Operating Procedure on the Use of Multiparametric Magnetic Resonance Imaging for the Diagnosis, Staging and Management of Prostate Cancer. *Journal of Urology* 2020;203(4):706–12. PMID: 31642740.

Briggs JG, Kim M, Gusev A, et al. Evaluation of In-Office MRI/US Fusion Transperineal Prostate Biopsy via Free-hand Device During Routine Clinical Practice. *Urology* 2021;155:26–32. PMID: 34048827.

Frye TP, George AK, Kilchevsky A, et al. Magnetic Resonance Imaging–Transrectal Ultrasound Guided Fusion Biopsy to Detect Progression in Patients with Existing Lesions on Active Surveillance for Low and Intermediate Risk Prostate Cancer. *Journal of Urology* 2017;197(3 Pt 1):640–46. PMID: 27613356.

Garnick M, Olumi A. Editorial Comment. *Urology* 2021;155:31–32. PMID: 34489003.

Jayadevan R, Felder ER, Kwan L, et al. Magnetic Resonance Imaging–Guided Confirmatory Biopsy for Initiating Active Surveillance of Prostate Cancer. *JAMA Network Open* 2019;2(9):e1911019. PMID: 31509206.

Kasivisvanathan V, Rannikko AS, Borghi M, et al. MRI-Targeted or Standard Biopsy for Prostate Cancer Diagnosis. *New England Journal of Medicine* 2018;378(19):1767–77. PMID: 29552975.

Klotz L, Chin J, Black PC, et al. Comparison of Multiparametric Magnetic Resonance Imaging–Targeted Biopsy with Systematic Transrectal Ultrasonography Biopsy for Biopsy-Naive Men at Risk for Prostate Cancer: A Phase 3 Randomized Clinical Trial. *JAMA Oncology* 2021;7(4):534–42. PMID: 33538782.

Pradere B, Veeratterapillay R, Dimitropoulos, K, et al. Nonantibiotic Strategies for the Prevention of Infectious Complications Following Prostate Biopsy: A Systematic Review and Meta-Analysis. *Journal of Urology* 2021;205(3):653–63. PMID: 33026903.

continued on page 53

It's now accepted practice to give antibiotics before and after transrectal biopsies to guard against infections, but they occur anyway—and, though still rare, serious infections from bacteria that can't be treated with conventional antibiotics are increasing. Strategies for reducing infections include cleansing the rectum with povidone-iodine (the same iodine solution you can buy at the drugstore) and enemas. Doctors can also culture bacteria obtained from a rectal swab to screen in advance for antibiotic-resistant strains. Targeting antibiotics to bacteria in the rectum has been proposed, but that approach has not been studied carefully.

Transperineal biopsy. An alternative to taking prostate biopsies through the rectum is to work through the perineum, the area between the anus and the base of the scrotum. With the transperineal approach, as it's called, the doctor, guided by ultrasound imaging, inserts the biopsy needle through cleaned perineal skin. A 2021 review of 90 clinical trials enrolling a combined 16,941 participants found that the risk of infectious complications is lower with transperineal biopsies than it is with biopsies given by the transrectal route. Because of that, transperineal biopsies are now favored in many countries. However, they have yet to be widely adopted in the United States, where the TRUS method still predominates.

Transperineal biopsies may be especially appropriate if antibiotic-resistant bacteria are detected in a rectal swab. And they are also done for patients who have had colon or rectal cancer surgery, for whom access through the rectum may be difficult.

In a 2015 study, investigators found that transperineal biopsies are better than standard TRUS biopsies at detecting high-grade tumors, and investigators who evaluated the feasibility of this approach at a single institution reported in 2021 that transperineal biopsies also detected tumors in the anterior (front) of the prostate that were not identified by pre-biopsy MRI. These tumors could potentially have been missed by a TRUS biopsy. However, just over 6% of the 130 men given transperineal biopsies during this study also had noninfectious complications, including blood clots and acute urinary retention.

This approach may also be used for a mapping biopsy (see Figure 10, page 77), when cancer has already been diagnosed and the surgeon plans to remove just the affected area of the prostate rather than the whole thing. However, transperineal biopsies are more painful and harder to perform than transrectal biopsies, and fewer urologists and radiologists are skilled in doing them.

MRI-guided biopsy. MRI scans generate detailed images of the prostate that can help doctors find cancers they might otherwise miss with ultrasound imaging. One promising approach is to take an MRI scan of the prostate before the biopsy and then, with computer software, fuse that high-resolution image with the real-time images generated by ultrasound during the biopsy procedure. Proponents say that these MRI-guided biopsies (also known as MRI-targeted or fusion-guided biopsies) can help doctors pinpoint suspicious areas better and thereby make the biopsies more accurate. In a consensus statement published in December 2016, the AUA and the Society of Abdominal Radiology asserted that men with suspected prostate cancer in whom TRUS biopsy found no cancer should undergo an MRI-guided biopsy.

Biopsy research

continued from page 52

Salami SS, Ben-Levi E, Yaskiv O, et al. In Patients with a Previous Negative Prostate Biopsy and a Suspicious Lesion on Magnetic Resonance Imaging, Is a 12-Core Biopsy Still Necessary in Addition to a Targeted Biopsy? *BJU International* 2015;115(4):562–70. PMID: 25252133.

Scott S, Samaratunga H, Chabert C, et al. Is Transperineal Prostate Biopsy More Accurate than Transrectal Biopsy in Determining Final Gleason Score and Clinical Risk Category? A Comparative Analysis. *BJU International* 2015;116(Suppl 3):26–30. PMID: 26260531.

Sidana A, Watson MJ, George AK, et al. Fusion Prostate Biopsy Outperforms 12-Core Systematic Prostate Biopsy in Patients with Prior Negative Systematic Biopsy: A Multi-Institutional Analysis. *Urologic Oncology* 2018;36(7):341.e1–e7. PMID: 29753548.

Biopsy complications

Derin O, Fonseca L, Sanchez-Salas R, et al. Infectious Complications of Prostate Biopsy: Winning Battles but Not War. *World Journal of Urology* 2020;38(11):2743–53. PMID: 32095882.

Liss MA, Ehdaie B, Loeb S, et al. An Update of the American Urological Association White Paper on the Prevention and Treatment of the More Common Complications Related to Prostate Biopsy. *Journal of Urology* 2017;198(2):329–34. PMID: 28363690.

Olvera-Posada D, Welk B, McLure JA, et al. A Population-Based Cohort Study of the Impact of Infectious Complications Requiring Hospitalization After Prostate Biopsy on Radical Prostatectomy Surgical Outcomes. *Urology* 2018;121:139–46. PMID: 30171923.

Queiroz MRG, Falsarella PM, Mariotti GC, et al. Comparison of Complications Rates Between Multiparametric Magnetic Resonance Imaging–Transrectal Ultrasound (TRUS) Fusion and Systematic TRUS Prostatic Biopsies. *Abdominal Radiology* 2019;44(2):732–38. PMID: 30255444.

PubMed See page 120.

Evidence published in 2018 further supports this recommendation. The researchers reviewed data from 779 men with persistently elevated PSA levels—suggesting that prostate cancer was present—but whose earlier TRUS biopsies were negative (that is, had not located any cancer). The men enrolled in the study each had an MRI-guided biopsy followed by a standard TRUS biopsy. In all, 346 cancers were detected, but the MRI-guided method found a higher proportion of high-grade tumors than the standard method did.

Experts are continuing to study how to use the MRI-guided approach to increase the likelihood of detecting cancer, and also how to determine which (if any) patients should be given this test first rather than as a follow-up after traditional biopsy. In 2021, for instance, investigators reported results from a clinical trial during which 453 men with elevated PSA were randomized to either a TRUS biopsy or to an MRI followed by MRI-guided biopsy of areas that looked suspicious for cancer. The findings showed that the MRI-guided and TRUS biopsies detected about the same number of clinically significant cancers. But fewer than half as many men in the MRI arm of the study wound up being diagnosed with low-grade cancers that are clinically insignificant. Furthermore, 83 of the 221 men given an MRI (37.5%) had a negative result and avoided a biopsy altogether. Additional studies with a longer follow-up are needed to confirm the results.

Other research suggests that in some cases, it may be better to use both methods together. In a 2020 study of 2,103 men, researchers detected 208 more cancers by performing both a standard biopsy and MRI-guided biopsy together than they did by giving standard biopsies alone. Importantly, 59 of those additional cancers were in high-risk categories. When given by itself, MRI-guided biopsy missed nearly 9% of high-grade cancers that were detected when both methods were used together.

In addition to using MRI-guided biopsy for cancer detection, doctors are beginning to use it to help select appropriate candidates for active surveillance, and then to monitor potential changes in the cancer that might require treatment.

Staging

If inspection of the biopsied tissue confirms prostate cancer, more tests may be ordered to find out if the cancer has spread to other parts of the body. Computed tomography (CT) or MRI techniques, which use x-rays and magnetic fields, respectively, can produce images that help doctors evaluate the spread of malignant cells to surrounding tissue, including the lymph nodes. A bone scan can reveal areas of bone that contain cancer. But these tests are not always accurate for detecting cancer that has spread beyond the prostate, and not all men need them, particularly if they have tumors with lower Gleason scores (see "How fast is it growing?" on page 56) and lower PSA levels. In some situations, however, doctors use them to help assign a stage to the cancer.

Ultimately, the prognosis and decisions about treatment depend on staging. A staging system is a common way of describing how far a cancer has progressed. There are different staging systems for prostate cancer, but the most widely used one is the TNM system, short for tumor-node-metastasis (see Figure 5, page 55). It describes the

continued on page 56

Figure 5. Stages of prostate cancer

The TNM system for classifying tumors (illustrated here) captures basic information about a cancer in a few letters and numbers—namely, the extent of the primary tumor (T), whether the cancer has spread to nearby lymph nodes (N), and whether it has spread to distant sites (M).

Stage T1

Your doctor can't feel these tumors during a DRE or see them with an imaging test such as a transrectal ultrasound.

- **T1a:** Tumor is found incidentally during transurethral resection of the prostate (TURP) for BPH; less than 5% of the tissue removed is cancerous, and is usually of low grade.
- **T1b:** Like T1a, but more than 5% of the tissue removed is cancerous or the cancer is high grade.
- **T1c (not shown):** Detected when an elevated PSA leads to a needle biopsy.

Stage T2

These cancers can be felt during a DRE and seem confined to the prostate.

- **T2a:** The cancer fills less than half of one side (left or right) of the prostate.
- **T2b:** Like T2a, but the cancer fills more than half of one side (left or right) of the prostate.
- **T2c (not shown):** Like T2a, but cancer is detected in both sides (left and right) of the prostate.

Stage T3

These cancers have broken through the prostate's fibrous capsule.

- **T3a:** The cancer extends outside the prostate, but has not spread to the seminal vesicles.
- **T3b:** The cancer has spread to the seminal vesicles.

Stage T4

Like T3 disease, but the cancer invades other nearby structures, such as the bladder or rectum.

Stages N and M

These cancers have metastasized to the pelvic lymph nodes (N1) or to other parts of the body (M1). Cancers that have spread to distant lymph nodes are classified as M1a, while cancers that have spread to the bones are M1b. Cancers that have spread to other sites—such as the lungs, but not the bones—are classified as M1c.

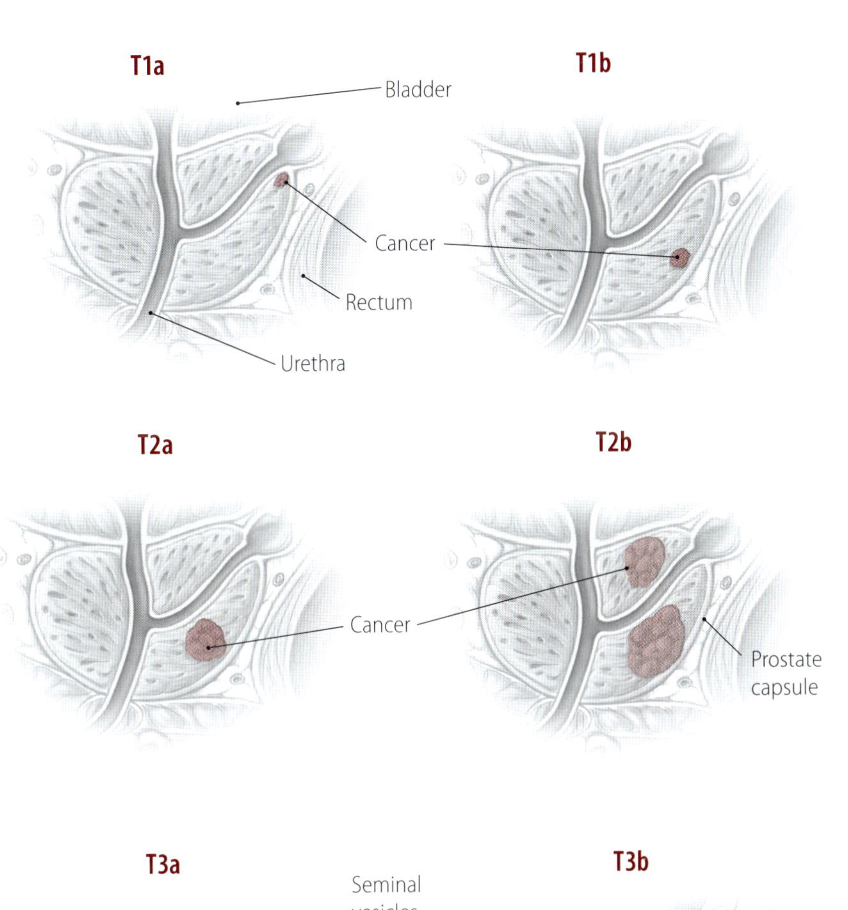

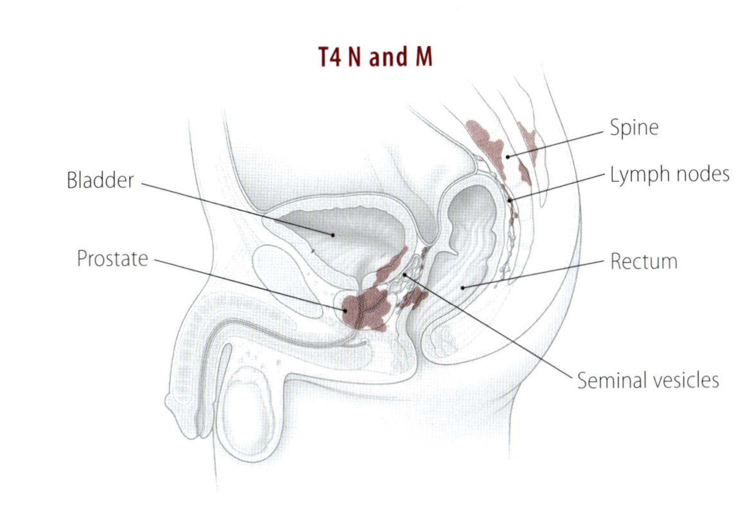

continued from page 54

extent of the primary tumor (T category), whether the cancer has spread to nearby lymph nodes (N category), and whether it has spread to distant sites (M category).

How fast is it growing?

Doctors use another assessment scale to predict the behavior of a prostate tumor, based on a microscopic evaluation of the biopsied tissue cells. A numerical grade, called the Gleason score, describes the cancer based on its aggressiveness and potential to spread (metastasize).

Tumors often consist of multiple types of cells (see Figure 6, below). Pathologists evaluate the most common type of cancer cell and assign a number to it. If these cells deviate only slightly from normal prostate tissue, they are likely to be slow-growing. In this case, the grade is Gleason 1. If they have changed to look more like cancer cells and are therefore likely to spread quickly to the bones or lymph nodes, the grade is Gleason 5, the highest rating. The same grading process is repeated for the second most common type of cell in the biopsy specimen.

Combining the two grades—4+3, for example—yields a Gleason score, which can range from 2 to 10. The higher the score, the faster the malignant cells are multiplying. Doctors assess Gleason scores not only for the tumor itself, but also for the surgical margins (the millimeter or two of tissue around the tumor that is also removed in order to make sure no cancer cells are left behind). If cancer cells are detected in the

Figure 6. Gleason patterns

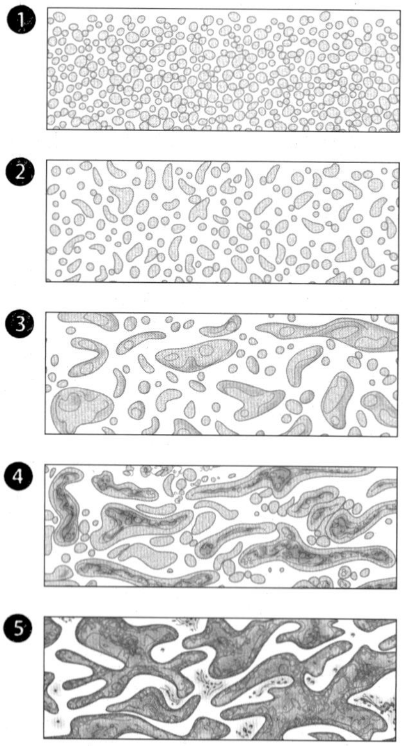

1 2 3 4 5

Well differentiated cells

Grade Group 1 (Gleason 3+3=6 or lower). Cells are small, of fairly uniform shape, and tightly packed together.

Grade Group 2 (Gleason 3+4=7). Cells display more varied and irregular shapes and are loosely packed.

Moderately differentiated cells

Grade Group 3 (Gleason 4+3=7). Cells are even more irregular in size and shape and are more dispersed; some cells are fused, and cell borders are less distinct.

Poorly differentiated cells

Grade Group 4 (Gleason 4+4=8). Many cells are fused into irregular masses; some cells (those darkly shaded) have begun to invade the connective tissue that separates cells.

Grade Group 5 (Gleason 4+5=9 or higher). Most of the tumor consists of irregular masses that have invaded the connective tissue.

surgical margins, high Gleason scores there can predict poor outcomes after surgery to remove the prostate (radical prostatectomy). Dr. Garnick considers giving radiation treatments after surgery if the margins contain any cells that score as Gleason pattern 4 or 5.

Though it's been widely adopted, the Gleason scoring system has some drawbacks. For instance, doctors today are debating whether tumors with a score lower than 3+3=6 should even be classified as cancer, given their indolent nature and the likelihood that they will never cause trouble. By the same token, the Gleason system makes a 3+3 tumor appear to be in the middle of the risk scale, when it's actually in the low-risk category. Moreover, since the first number in the system carries more weight than the second, a Gleason 4+3=7 tumor is actually more dangerous than a Gleason 3+4=7 tumor, even though the final scores for each are the same.

To simplify matters, scientists have adopted a five-tier grading system that ranks tumors from Grade Group 1 (the least dangerous) to Grade Group 5 (the most dangerous). Using this approach, a Gleason 3+4=7 tumor is classified Grade Group 2, while a Gleason 4+3=7 tumor is classified Grade Group 3. The new system also distinguishes more clearly between high-grade cancers that would traditionally be scored as Gleason 8, 9, and 10. A study published in 2016 found that Grade Group 5 tumors ordinarily described as Gleason 9 or 10 were actually twice as hazardous as Grade Group 4 tumors scored otherwise as Gleason 8. (For reference, see "Alternative to Gleason scoring," at right.)

The new system has some obvious benefits: the grade stratification is more accurate, and it's also less likely to lead to overtreatment. That's because men diagnosed with Grade Group 1 cancer might be less anxious to begin treatment than men who've been assigned a Gleason score of 6 out of 10, even though it is the same grade.

Alternative to Gleason scoring

Epstein JI, Zelefsky MJ, Sjoberg DD, et al. A Contemporary Prostate Cancer Grading System: A Validated Alternative to the Gleason Score. *European Urology* 2016;69(3):428–35. PMID: 26166626.

PubMed See page 120.

Active surveillance

Some men diagnosed with prostate cancer need no treatment: for example, a man with a small, slowly progressing stage T1 cancer with a Gleason score of 5 or 6 who also has another serious medical condition, or a man with a life expectancy of less than 10 years. Prostate cancers often take 15 to 20 years, or even more, to grow to a detectable size and cause symptoms; in the meantime, they cause little harm. Many older men, especially those over age 75, are more likely to die of another condition before their prostate cancer becomes troublesome or dangerous, and they may face greater risks from surgery or other treatments than from the cancer itself.

At the other end of the spectrum are younger men—those ages 50 to 60, with an aggressive cancer in the early stages and a family history of prostate cancer. Virtually all doctors agree that these men require treatment, despite the lack of convincing information on whether treatment improves either overall survival or cancer-specific survival in these cases. Treatment might also make sense for men suffering from BPH, because removing the prostate through surgery—or reducing its size with other therapies—not only treats the cancer but also may improve urinary symptoms.

But a significant number of men fall into a gray area, where the decision of whether or not to treat isn't clear-cut. Although estimates vary, 40% of men diagnosed

Active surveillance vs. watchful waiting

In the past, doctors used the term "watchful waiting" to describe any strategy that involved following a prostate tumor to see if it worsened. Testing was done not on a set schedule, but only when symptoms developed or worsened. And while some patients eventually had their cancer treated, others had no intention of doing so.

Today, patients who monitor their cancer closely and plan to have treatment when its activity increases are said to be pursuing active surveillance. Many doctors now reserve the terms "watchful waiting" and "observation" for cases in which patients don't plan to have treatment for prostate cancer because of their age or health.

Active surveillance

Bloom JB, Daneshvar MA, Lebastchi AH, et al. Risk of Adverse Pathology at Prostatectomy in the Era of MRI and Targeted Biopsies; Rethinking Active Surveillance for Intermediate Risk Prostate Cancer Patients. *Urologic Oncology* 2021;39(10):729.e1–e6. PMID: 33736975.

Cooperberg MR, Carroll PR. Trends in Management for Patients with Localized Prostate Cancer, 1990–2013. *JAMA* 2015;314(1):80–82. PMID: 26151271.

Deka R, Courtney PT, Parsons JK, et al. Association Between African American Race and Clinical Outcomes in Men Treated for Low-Risk Prostate Cancer with Active Surveillance. *JAMA* 2020;324(17):1747–54. PMID: 33141207.

Detsky JS, Ghiam AF, Mamedov A, et al. Impact of Biopsy Compliance on Outcomes for Patients on Active Surveillance for Prostate Cancer. *Journal of Urology* 2020;204(5):934–40. PMID: 32330406.

continued on page 59

with prostate cancer—as many as 100,000 Americans each year—have tumors that are so small and apparently slow-growing that they meet the criteria for active surveillance. This is a strategy that involves monitoring the cancer closely (with prostate biopsies, DREs, PSA tests, and imaging scans as needed) and choosing to start treatment when and if it advances or shows evidence of increasing activity. Other names for active surveillance include expectant management, active monitoring, and active surveillance with delayed intent to treat (see "Active surveillance vs. watchful waiting," at left).

Studies have shown that men on active surveillance for low-risk cancer report significantly better urinary function, sexual function, and sexual satisfaction than men who had chosen surgery or radiation therapy. A 2018 study found that while patients are likely to have initial worries about future prospects for their cancer when they first go on active surveillance, their cancer-specific stress and anxiety levels also decrease significantly with time if monitoring shows the disease is remaining stable.

Because Black men are at higher risk of aggressive prostate cancer and recurrence after treatment than are whites—and because favorable outcomes with active surveillance have mainly been documented in white populations—Black men were advised for years to approach active surveillance cautiously. Mounting evidence, however, shows that they have results similar to those of white men if given access to the same quality of care. The authors of a 2021 review of 12 published studies concluded that even though Black men have an increased risk of progression, the risk is not so great that they should be discouraged from active surveillance. Along those lines, a 2020 study found that Black and white men on active surveillance had nearly identical rates of metastasis (1.5% and 1.4%, respectively) and death from prostate cancer (1.1% and 1.0%) after nearly eight years of follow-up.

Indeed, the increase in active surveillance has been accompanied by growing evidence of its long-term safety, especially for men with low-risk prostate cancer (see Table 4, page 59, for the classification of risks). A study by U.S. researchers published in 2015 showed that 93% of men with low-risk disease were still alive 10 years after being put on active surveillance, and nearly 70% of them were still alive after 15 years. A 2020 update on the same group of men found that after all this time since starting active surveillance, the risk of dying from prostate cancer or developing metastatic disease was only 0.1%, although half the men eventually wound up having surgery or radiation therapy.

Similarly, a Canadian study, first reported in 2015, found that only 1.5% of 993 men put on active surveillance in 1995 (a total of 15 men) had died from prostate cancer two decades later. However, differences emerged among the men with low- and intermediate-risk disease. The following year, the investigators reported that 30 of the men ultimately developed metastases, and 28 of those were in the intermediate-risk group. The authors placed the 15-year risk of metastases at 15% to 20% for this group—but close to zero for men in the low-risk group. Experts emphasize that some intermediate-risk patients may still make good candidates for active surveillance, but that caution should be exercised when making that decision. The Canadian study was in the process of being updated in 2021, and results were not available as we went to

Table 4. Criteria for classifying prostate cancer as low, intermediate, or high risk

Risk	PSA level		Gleason score		Cancer stage
Low	under 10 ng/ml	and	3+3	and	T1–2a
Intermediate	10–20 ng/ml	and/or	3+4 or 4+3	and/or	T2b–2c
High	over 20 ng/ml	and/or	4+4 or higher	and/or	T3+

Source: D'Amico AV. Risk-Based Management of Prostate Cancer. *New England Journal of Medicine* 2011;365(2):169–71. PMID: 21751910.

press. However, in 2020, the Canadian team did publish one preliminary finding from its ongoing analysis. It showed an increasing risk of metastases among men who don't stick with their scheduled biopsies. The authors cited missed windows of opportunity for detecting worsening cancer before it begins to spread. (For references, see "Active surveillance," page 58.)

Criteria for active surveillance

Active surveillance is most often considered in cases of prostate cancer that are considered low or very low in risk. The criteria for determining which cases are eligible for active surveillance are not uniform or strict. Several research groups and medical centers have developed their own standards. But the important elements of commonly used criteria include the following:

- PSA less than 10 ng/ml
- Gleason score equal to or less than 6
- tumor stage of T1c (typically found by PSA testing) or T2a (a small nodule that can be felt during a DRE).

A man's age and health also should be factored in to the active surveillance decision. All other things being equal, the older a man with low-risk prostate cancer is, the more suitable he is for active surveillance, because it's likely that other health conditions will cause illness and death before his prostate cancer would. In 2019, researchers reported results showing that active surveillance can also be suitable for younger men with low-risk cancers, meaning that the men have PSA levels below 10 ng/ml at the outset and their tumors are Grade Group 1 (Gleason 3+3 or lower). After six years of follow-up, the researchers detected no difference in survival among men who began active surveillance for low-risk prostate cancer before age 60 versus later in life.

In 2018, the National Comprehensive Cancer Network issued updated clinical guidelines, stating that while active surveillance is preferable for men in lower risk categories, it also may be considered for men with "favorable" intermediate-risk prostate cancer, who are defined as being in Grade Groups 1 or 2, with Gleason scores no higher than 3+4=7, PSA in the range of 10–20 ng/ml, and having detectable cancer in fewer than half of their biopsy cores. New research indicates that MRI-guided biopsies given together with TRUS biopsies are better at finding suitable intermediate-risk can-

Active surveillance

continued from page 58

Gökce MI, Sundi D, Schaeffer E, et al. Is Active Surveillance a Suitable Option for African American Men with Prostate Cancer? A Systematic Literature Review. *Prostate Cancer and Prostatic Diseases* 2017;20(2):127–36. PMID: 28417980.

Lonergan PE, Jeong CW, Washington SL, et al. Active Surveillance in Intermediate-Risk Prostate Cancer with PSA 10–20 ng/mL: Pathological Outcome Analysis of a Population-Level Database. *Prostate Cancer and Prostatic Diseases* 2021;Electronic publication ahead of print. PMID: 34508180.

Mahal BA, Butler S, Franco I, et al. Use of Active Surveillance or Watchful Waiting for Low-Risk Prostate Cancer and Management Trends Across Risk Groups in the United States, 2010–2015. *JAMA* 2019;321(7):704–06. PMID: 30743264.

Marzouk K, Assel M, Ehdaie B, et al. Long-Term Cancer Specific Anxiety in Men Undergoing Active Surveillance of Prostate Cancer: Findings From a Large Prospective Cohort. *Journal of Urology* 2018;200(6):1250–55. PMID: 29886089.

Salari K, Kuppermann D, Preston MA, et al. Active Surveillance of Prostate Cancer Is a Viable Option for Men Younger than 60 Years. *Journal of Urology* 2019;201(4):721–27. PMID: 30664083.

Tosoian JJ, Mamawala M, Epstein JI. Intermediate and Longer-Term Outcomes from a Prospective Active-Surveillance Program for Favorable-Risk Prostate Cancer. *Journal of Clinical Oncology* 2015;33(30):3379–85. PMID: 26324359.

continued on page 60

PubMed See page 120.

Active surveillance
continued from page 59

Tosoian JJ, Mamawala M, Epstein JI, et al. Active Surveillance of Grade Group 1 Prostate Cancer: Long-term Outcomes from a Large Prospective Cohort. *European Urology* 2020;77(6):675–82. PMID: 31918957.

Vigneswaran HT, Mittelstaedt L, Crippa A, et al. Progression on Active Surveillance for Prostate Cancer in Black Men: A Systematic Review and Meta-Analysis. *Prostate Cancer and Prostatic Diseases* 2021;Electronic publication ahead of print. PMID: 34239046.

Yamamoto T, Musunuru HB, Vesprini D, et al. Metastatic Prostate Cancer in Men Initially Treated with Active Surveillance. *Journal of Urology* 2016;195(5):1409–14. PMID: 26707510.

didates than TRUS biopsies by themselves. But men in this group should be selected and monitored carefully. For a 2021 study, investigators analyzed prostate tissue samples from men who had surgery to remove the prostate after having been on active surveillance. They found that men who had been diagnosed with "favorable" intermediate-risk tumors were more likely to have high-grade cancer in the samples than men who had been diagnosed with low-risk prostate tumors. Still, active surveillance rates are increasing steadily for intermediate-risk as well as low-risk prostate cancer, according to study results published in 2019. The percentage of men with low-risk tumors who chose active surveillance in the United States jumped from 14.5% in 2010 to 42.1% in 2015, and the percentage of men with intermediate-risk cancer who chose active surveillance increased from 5.8% to 9.6% over the same period. (For references, see "Active surveillance," page 57.)

Monitoring during active surveillance

During active surveillance, it's important to undergo regular monitoring to determine if the cancer has become more aggressive. If it has, it's time to consider treatment.

Monitoring recommendations vary. At a minimum, monitoring should consist of regular DREs to assess tumor growth and periodic PSA tests to check for increases in blood levels that might indicate a progression of the cancer. These follow-up tests

What do the studies show about treatment vs. observation?

For low-risk cancer, surgery does not help men live longer than active surveillance, according to various observational studies (studies that do not randomize patients to a particular treatment, but analyze outcomes after people make their own choices). However, two important randomized controlled trials comparing surgery and observation have delivered a split verdict.

PIVOT. The Prostate Cancer Intervention Versus Observation Trial (PIVOT) was a federally funded randomized controlled trial comparing surgery with observation. The results, published in 2012, showed that after 12 years of follow-up, radical prostatectomy did not improve chances of surviving any more than watchful waiting.

The PIVOT researchers decided before the trial to classify participants by risk (determined by a combination of PSA results, Gleason score, and tumor stage). They found that while surgery had no benefit for men with low-risk prostate cancer, it did appear to improve survival in men with high-risk tumors, although the number of men in that group was too small for the results to be definitive.

It's worth noting that about 30% of the men in PIVOT were Blacks, who have been underrepresented in clinical trials of all types. The outcomes for Blacks did not differ from those of the rest of the men in the study.

The PIVOT study had two important limitations. First, it fell well short of the enrollment goal of 2,000 participants, so some researchers have questioned whether PIVOT was large enough to provide definitive conclusions. Second, the average age of the men who were enrolled was 67, so reduced life expectancy might explain why men were most likely to die of causes other than prostate cancer.

SPCG-4. In contrast to the PIVOT study, the Scandinavian Prostate Cancer Group Study 4 (SPCG-4) concluded that radical prostatectomy does improve men's odds of surviving. Between 1989 and 1999, SPCG-4 enrolled 695 men in Sweden, Finland, and Iceland who were randomly assigned to radical prostatectomy or watchful waiting. By 2017, 77% (261 men) of those assigned to surgery had died, compared with 83% (292 men) in the watchful waiting group. More importantly, 71 of the 261 deaths in the surgery group were specifically from prostate cancer, compared with 110 out of 292 deaths in the watchful waiting group.

It is questionable, though, how applicable the SPCG-4 results are to American men today. The men recruited to the SPCG-4 study were diagnosed not on the basis of a PSA test (as is common in the United States) but because of symptoms such as pain or difficulty urinating. This means that their cancers were probably more advanced than those detected through PSA screening. In addition, the study's watchful waiting group did not involve the type of monitoring now recommended for men undergoing active surveillance.

should be scheduled every four to 12 months, depending on a man's age, biopsy results, and anxiety level.

In addition, biopsies are generally done every one to three years. Some guidelines recommend annual biopsies. But a number of experts, including Dr. Garnick, believe that annual prostate biopsies shouldn't be recommended automatically, because they can lead to complications, including erectile dysfunction, infection, and other problems. Moreover, other tests can provide key information without subjecting a man to a biopsy. Multiparametric MRI (see "Special MRI imaging techniques," page 50) might generate information about the cancer that makes some biopsies unnecessary, especially when combined with repeated PSA measures and other tests such as the PHI and the 4Kscore (see "Variations on the PSA test," page 48).

Optimal timing for repeat biopsies remains an ongoing area of research. A study published in 2020 indicates that some men may not need biopsies as often as others. The researchers compared outcomes in 1,400 men with low-risk prostate cancer who had been on active surveillance for four years. Men with the greatest number of positive biopsy cores at diagnosis as well as higher PSA levels that also rose faster over time were most likely to have worsening disease. (For reference, see "Monitoring for active surveillance," above right.) For such men, more frequent biopsies are warranted. Dr. Garnick integrates information from genetic testing, previous biopsies, and MRI

Monitoring for active surveillance

Cooperberg MR, Zheng Y, Faino AV, et al. Tailoring Intensity of Active Surveillance for Low-Risk Prostate Cancer Based on Individualized Prediction of Risk Stability. *JAMA Oncology* 2020;6(10):e204187. PMID: 32852532.

PubMed See page 120.

Additional studies. In the United Kingdom, the Prostate Testing for Cancer and Treatment (ProtecT) study randomly assigned more than 1,500 men to either surgery, external beam radiation, or active monitoring. Ten-year results reported in 2016 found no differences in overall survival among the three groups. Metastases developed more often in the active monitoring group. It may be that the metastases occurred predominantly in men with intermediate-risk prostate cancer, but this was not reported.

In 2015, two observational studies showed increasing evidence for the safety of active surveillance for men with low-risk disease, though these two studies did not compare these men against patients who underwent surgery. An update of one of those studies published in 2020 showed that the risk of cancer death or metastasis among 1,818 men monitored on active surveillance for up to 15 years was less than 1%.

Data are also being collected through an international Web-based registry for the Prostate Cancer Research International: Active Surveillance (PRIAS) study. Ten-year results, published in 2016, showed that 60% of 5,302 men from 18 countries eventually switched over from surveillance to treatment, based on the number of biopsy samples that contained cancer (three or more positive biopsies compared with just one or two) and PSA density, which is the PSA level divided by the volume of the prostate.

Sources: Bill-Axelson A, Holmberg L, Garmo H, et al. Radical Prostatectomy or Watchful Waiting in Prostate Cancer—29-Year Follow-Up. *New England Journal of Medicine* 2018;379(24):2319–29. PMID: 30575473.

Donovan JL, Hamdy FC, Lane JA, et al. Patient-Reported Outcomes After Monitoring, Surgery, or Radiotherapy for Prostate Cancer. *New England Journal of Medicine* 2016;375(15):1425–37. PMID: 27626365.

Hamdy FC, Donovan, JL, Lane JA, et al. 10-Year Outcomes After Monitoring, Surgery, or Radiotherapy for Localized Prostate Cancer. *New England Journal of Medicine* 2016;375(15):1415–24. PMID: 27626136.

Klotz L, Vesprini D, Sethukavalan P, et al. Long-Term Follow-Up of a Large Active Surveillance Cohort of Patients with Prostate Cancer. *Journal of Clinical Oncology* 2015;33(3):272–77. PMID: 25512465.

Tosoian JJ, Mamawala M, Epstein JI. Intermediate and Longer-Term Outcomes from a Prospective Active-Surveillance Program for Favorable-Risk Prostate Cancer. *Journal of Clinical Oncology* 2015;33(30):3379–85. PMID: 26324359.

Tosoian JJ, Mamawala M, Epstein JI, et al. Active Surveillance of Grade Group 1 Prostate Cancer: Long-Term Outcomes from a Large Prospective Cohort. *European Urology* 2020;77(6):675–82. PMID: 31918957.

Wilt TJ, Brawer MK, Jones KM, et al. Radical Prostatectomy Versus Observation for Localized Prostate Cancer. *New England Journal of Medicine* 2012;367(3):203–13. PMID: 22808955.

to determine whether it's possible to lengthen the interval between biopsies to reduce the risk for complications or the need for continued biopsies.

That said, there's no question that regular monitoring of some kind is necessary while you are on active surveillance; without it, you run the risk that the cancer may grow and spread to a stage that makes it much more difficult to treat. Once on active surveillance, men should stick with their monitoring plan. If PSA readings increase sharply or if the doctor feels a new lump during a DRE, the cancer may be advancing, and treatment can be reconsidered. A change in urinary habits can also signal that it's time to begin treatment.

Signs that it may be time to consider treatment

Men on active surveillance can change their minds and, in consultation with a doctor, opt for treatment. They are not locked in.

But more often, a treatment recommendation is triggered when a low-risk cancer begins to exhibit features of an intermediate- or high-risk one. Active surveillance hasn't been standardized, and recommendations for exactly what should trigger a treatment recommendation vary. Most doctors would recommend treatment in the following circumstances:

- The Gleason score on a follow-up biopsy is equal to or greater than 7, especially if the primary score is a Gleason pattern 4.
- PSA doubling time accelerates.
- There is increased evidence of disease, such as finding more cores with cancer during a follow-up biopsy or discovering that the percentage of cancerous cells in individual cores is increasing.
- Significant changes are noted during a DRE.
- Significant changes are noted on a multiparametric MRI scan.
- You have a change in urinary habits. The doctor will need to determine if the cause is BPH or cancer (or both).

Treating prostate cancer

One thing is certain about prostate cancer: it's complicated—very complicated. Often there is no obvious choice when it comes to treatment, and you will need to weigh your options carefully and base your decision, with the help of your doctor and your loved ones, on many factors—not only the stage of your cancer, but also your age, lifestyle, and risk of side effects such as urinary incontinence and erectile dysfunction. You might even opt for no treatment at all, preferring active surveillance.

If you choose treatment, there are several initial options: radical prostatectomy (surgically removing the prostate gland); radiation, including external beam or implanted pellets (brachytherapy); focal therapy (which leaves most of the gland intact); or hormonal therapy (which suppresses testosterone, a hormonal "fuel" for prostate cancer). Each of these treatments has pluses and minuses, and despite years of research and efforts to improve results, complication rates remain stubbornly high.

That's especially true in the case of sexual complications. Men often report difficulty achieving erections for one to two years after radical prostatectomy, even when surgeons try to avoid damaging the nerves and blood vessels in the prostate that control erectile functioning. Sexual complication rates tend to be lower with radiation than they are with surgery, but radiation is associated with higher rates of long-term urinary incontinence and irritation, and impotence rates also tend to rise with time.

Prostate cancer treatments therefore involve complex trade-offs. They can be used alone or in combination, depending on a man's age, the stage of the cancer, and personal preferences regarding the side effects of the treatments and the lifestyle changes they may entail.

Numerous medications have been approved over the past 15 years. Among them:

- abiraterone (Zytiga),* cabazitaxel (Jevtana), and sipuleucel-T (Provenge) for men with advanced cancer
- apalutamide (Erleada) and darolutamide (Nubeqa) for men with advanced prostate cancer who no longer respond to first-line hormonal therapy
- degarelix (Firmagon),* a hormonal therapy drug
- denosumab (Xgeva) for bone complications of prostate cancer treatment
- enzalutamide (Xtandi)* for men with advanced cancer
- olaparib (Lynparza) for men with advanced prostate cancer who no longer respond to hormonal therapy or chemotherapy and who have mutations in BRCA1, BRCA2, or other DNA repair genes
- pembrolizumab (Keytruda) for patients who test positive for microsatellite instability and mismatch repair mutations (microsatellite instability refers to a predisposition toward gene mutations resulting from faulty DNA mismatch repair)
- rucaparib (Rubraca) for men with advanced prostate cancer who no longer respond to either enzalutamide or abiraterone and have either inherited or acquired mutations in BRCA1 and BRCA2
- radium-223 (Xofigo) for men with advanced prostate cancer and metastases to the bones but not other organs
- relugolix (Orgovyx)* for men with advanced prostate cancer.

__Editor's note:__ Dr. Marc Garnick, editor in chief of the Annual, *previously served as a consultant to Ferring Pharmaceuticals, the manufacturer of degarelix. He also served as an expert on patent issues related to abiraterone and enzalutamide and has served on a scientific board for Myovant, the manufacturer of relugolix.*

The wide variety of treatments can be confusing for patients and doctors alike. But it isn't simply a question of variety. No one treatment has emerged as preferred. Guidelines from the National Comprehensive Cancer Network can help with decision making. With this in mind, the following sections describe the available treatments, with the aim of helping you make a decision based on your doctor's recommendations and how a particular treatment will likely affect your quality of life.

Surgery

The best candidates for surgery are men whose disease is confined to the gland itself (stages T1 and T2), who are under age 70, and who are in good general health. Sur-

Prostate cancer surgery

Agrawal V, Xiaoyue M, Hu JC, et al. Trends in Diagnosis and Disparities in Initial Management of High-Risk Prostate Cancer in the US. *JAMA Network Open* 2020;3(8):e2014674. PMID: 32865572.

Costello AJ. Considering the Role of Radical Prostatectomy in 21st Century Prostate Cancer Care. *Nature Reviews Urology* 2020;17(3):177–88. PMID: 32086498.

gery that removes the entire prostate gland is called radical prostatectomy, and it's long been the standard surgical treatment for prostate cancer. In this context, radical has nothing to do with politics. It means removing affected tissue and any surrounding tissue that might also be affected. For example, a radical prostatectomy almost always involves removing the seminal vesicles, slender saclike glands that, along with the prostate, release fluid that becomes part of semen. In most cases, the surgeon also removes pelvic lymph nodes. Radical prostatectomy was once offered routinely to men with low-risk prostate cancer. Today, this type of surgery is reserved mostly for men with intermediate- and high-risk prostate cancer, while those with lower-risk tumors are generally treated with other techniques or followed with active surveillance. (For general references on surgery, see "Prostate cancer surgery," at left.)

Over the years, however, the way this surgery is performed has undergone a profound shift. In the traditional technique, called radical retropubic prostatectomy, the surgeon would make an incision from just below the navel to the pubic bone to gain access to the prostate. This open surgical technique has been supplanted by laparoscopic surgery—which involves inserting instruments and tiny cameras through much smaller "keyhole" incisions—and in particular by robot-assisted laparoscopic surgery. In robot-assisted surgery, the surgeon sits at a console and uses remote controls to move robotic arms that are holding laparoscopic instruments (see Figure 7, below).

The use of robotic surgery for prostate cancer has skyrocketed since its approval by the FDA in 2000; by 2014, it accounted for up to 90% of radical prostatectomies

Figure 7. Operating robotically

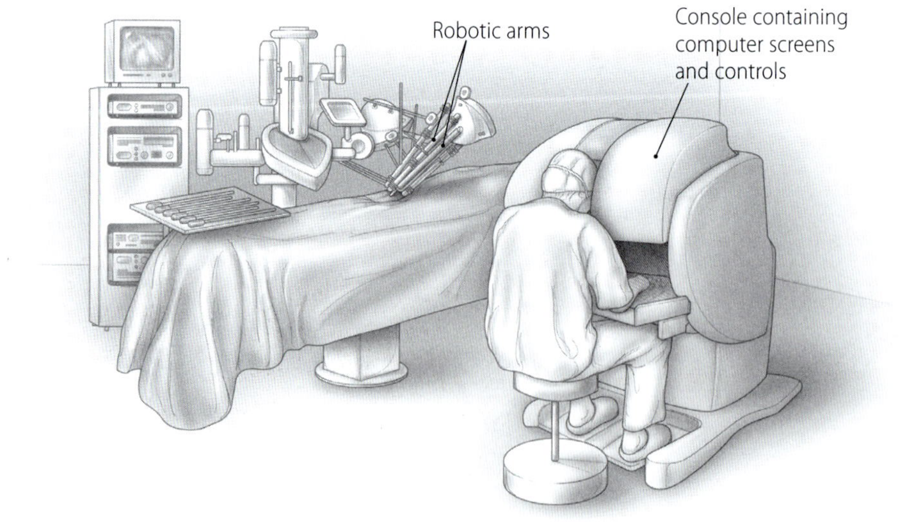

To perform a robot-assisted laparoscopic prostatectomy, the surgeon sits at a console several feet away from the operating table and manipulates robotic arms fitted with tiny cameras and surgical instruments to locate and remove the diseased prostate gland. The console contains two full-color computer screens that provide a magnified, three-dimensional view of the prostate and surrounding tissues. The surgeon guides the robotic arms by manipulating the controls while watching the screens.

performed in the United States. As surgeons have gained more experience with robotic surgery, the risks associated with it have fallen. Patients treated with robotic surgery often have less blood loss, less pain, and shorter recovery time than patients treated with traditional methods. However, several international studies comparing the experience of patients treated with either robotic or traditional approaches showed no difference in cancer outcomes, continence, or sexual functioning. (For references, see "Robotic surgery research," at right.)

Still, study after study has shown that the most important determinant of surgical success is the experience and skill of the surgeon, not whether the surgery is open or robotic. The best results, in terms of avoiding complications such as urinary incontinence, are obtained by surgeons who do large numbers of these procedures in high-volume hospitals.

Leaving no cancer behind

Before taking out the prostate—except in the case of the perineal technique (see "Another surgical option," page 66)—the surgeon may remove lymph nodes that could have been infiltrated by the cancer. A pathologist will immediately examine the lymph nodes. If cancer is present, the operation usually will go no further because this means the cancer has spread beyond the prostate, in which case other treatments are more appropriate than removing the prostate. Some surgeons advocate going ahead with the prostatectomy anyway. For that reason, it's important to discuss this possibility ahead of time with your surgeon, so that you can express your preference about whether to go forward with the prostatectomy.

If the lymph nodes show no cancer, the surgeon carefully separates the prostate and the seminal vesicles from the surrounding tissues and removes them. Later, the pathologist examines these organs. If the cancer is confined to the prostate, it likely won't return. If the cancer has already spread beyond the capsule surrounding the gland, additional treatment may be necessary.

Nerve-sparing (anatomic) surgery

Men have traditionally shuddered at the risks of radical prostatectomy, especially permanent impotence, which used to occur in nearly all cases. But that began to change in the early 1980s, when nerve-sparing surgery (also called anatomic prostate cancer surgery) was developed. During this surgery, doctors spare the two bundles of nerves that lie on either side of the prostate gland and control erections. This type of operation may also reduce the likelihood of other serious side effects, such as urinary incontinence and significant blood loss.

Almost all men undergoing prostatectomy would prefer to have the nerve-sparing procedure, and it's available across the country. However, success is not guaranteed. If the tumor is too close to a nerve bundle, the nerves can't be saved—and saving one nerve bundle is not as likely to preserve erectile function as saving both of them. Even if the procedure is successful, it can take a year or more for the tiny nerve fibers—which often stop transmitting impulses when they've been traumatized by the surgery—to heal sufficiently to restore sexual function.

Robotic surgery research

Arenas-Gallo C, Shoag JE, Hu JC. Optimizing Surgical Techniques in Robot-Assisted Radical Prostatectomy. *Urologic Clinics of North America* 2021;48(1):1–9. PMID: 33218583.

Coughlin GD, Yaxley JW, Chambers SK, et al. Robot-Assisted Laparoscopic Prostatectomy Versus Open Radical Retropubic Prostatectomy: 24-Month Outcomes from a Randomised Controlled Study. *Lancet Oncology* 2018;19(8):1051–60. PMID: 30017351.

Gershman B, Psutka SP, McGovern FJ, et al. Patient-Reported Functional Outcomes Following Open, Laparoscopic, and Robotic Assisted Radical Prostatectomy Performed by High-Volume Surgeons at High-Volume Hospitals. *European Urology Focus* 2016;2(2):172–79. PMID: 28723533.

Kumar A, Samavedi S, Bates AS, et al. Safety of Selective Nerve Sparing in High Risk Prostate Cancer During Robot-Assisted Radical Prostatectomy. *Journal of Robotic Surgery* 2017;11(2):129–38. PMID: 27435701.

Preisser F, Nazzani S, Mazzone E, et al. Comparison of Open Versus Robotically Assisted Cytoreductive Radical Prostatectomy for Metastatic Prostate Cancer. *Clinical Genitourinary Cancer* 2019;17(5):e939–94. PMID: 31375352.

Tholomier C, Couture F, Ajib K, et al. Oncological and Functional Outcomes of a Large Canadian Robotic-Assisted Radical Prostatectomy Database with 10 Years of Surgical Experience. *Canadian Journal of Urology* 2019;26(4):9843–51. PMID: 31469640.

PubMed See page 120.

> **Another surgical option**
>
> The perineal technique for radical prostatectomy involves the surgeon gaining access to the prostate by making an incision in the perineum, the area between the anus and the base of the scrotum. Proponents of this approach say that it causes less pain. However, it is seldom used. The big disadvantage is that it doesn't permit access to the pelvic lymph nodes, where prostate cancer may have spread, and so a separate operation or incision may be required to access the nodes.
>
> As noted earlier, the transparineal approach is also used for biopsies (see "Transperineal biosy," page 53).

Estimates of the number of men undergoing radical prostatectomy who actually regain their ability to have erections range widely, from 13% to 57%. Why the enormous range? It's at least partly because some research relies on patients' reports, while other research relies on physicians' estimates. Patients are often reluctant to tell their doctors about such problems unless they are specifically asked about them.

It's important to choose an experienced surgeon. Recovery of sexual function also depends on the patient's age and the location of the tumor. Medication may be prescribed to help this process (see "Treating erectile dysfunction," page 104).

Recovery

Depending on the technique used and a man's health, recovery usually involves one to three days in the hospital and several weeks at home. Men undergoing robotic surgery tend to go home faster than those undergoing open surgery. The patient will need to urinate through a catheter for a week or two while the urethra heals.

Complications

Erectile dysfunction and urinary incontinence are the most common—and often most distressing—complications of prostatectomy. For a 2020 study, researchers compared long-term outcomes in 2,005 men ages 59 to 70 who selected surgery, radiation, or active surveillance for localized prostate cancer. Among the surgically treated men, 61% on average were still reporting erections insufficient for sexual intercourse five years later. Other research shows that most men develop some degree of incontinence requiring use of a pad, with 15% to 20% of patients developing severe cases. Although these common side effects aren't always permanent, recovery can take several years. Researchers contacted more than 3,000 men who had a radical prostatectomy between 2007 and 2013. More than half the men claimed to have recovered good urinary functioning within two to three years. And between 30% and 40% said they could achieve erections within the same time frame.

The likelihood of a successful outcome—in terms of preserving potency, preventing incontinence, and most importantly, curing the cancer—generally correlates with the surgeon's experience. The number of procedures a surgeon performs does not necessarily make him or her better than one who does fewer; however, a minimum of 15 to 20 prostatectomies per year is necessary to be sufficiently skilled at the operation. A man's sexual potency before surgery can also predict his capacity to achieve erections afterward. Most men who report good sexual potency before surgery can achieve normal erections within two years, while recovery rates among those who report poor initial potency are far lower over the same time period. A man's age and weight also factor into how long it takes him to recover his sexual potency, along with the experience of the surgeon performing his operation. A 2019 study with 2,364 men found that potency recovery rates have actually been declining for 10 years. But the authors pointed out that could be because more men are having prostate cancer surgery when they're older and have other health problems that can slow their recovery down. (For references, see "Outcomes of prostate cancer surgery," page 67.) From personal experience, Dr. Garnick has found that men with poor erectile functioning before radical prostatectomy are unlikely to return to baseline potency after surgery. His experience also shows that most men do not regain baseline potency after surgery that preserves only one of the two nerve bundles. By contrast, men who have good potency before surgery and whose surgery preserves both of the nerve bundles have reasonable chances of recovering erectile function.

Radiation therapy

Radiation is a reasonable alternative to surgery for certain prostate cancers, particularly for localized cancer (cancer that is still confined to the prostate gland). It can be delivered to the prostate in two ways: by aiming an external beam of radiation at the tumor or by surgically implanting small radioactive pellets in the prostate gland (an approach called brachytherapy). As with surgery, no single form of radiation therapy has emerged as the "winner." Moreover, within those two big categories of external beam radiation and brachytherapy, there are many variations and modifications. Table 5, page 68, will help you compare them.

If you choose radiation treatment, your doctor will likely recommend a treatment approach that takes into account your risk profile. In men with low- or intermediate-risk cancer, radiation will be directed to the entire prostate plus the seminal vesicles. In men with higher-risk cancer, the pelvic lymph nodes may be radiated as well. The criteria for low-, intermediate-, and high-risk cancer vary, depending on the study, the doctor, and the medical center. Table 4, page 59, gives one commonly used set of criteria. Online risk calculators can be very helpful and are relatively easy to understand. However, the best way to assess your risk is to work with your doctor.

Radiation vs. surgery

Whether to opt for surgery or radiation is a complicated decision informed by many different variables, including age, personal preferences, and the presence or absence of other accompanying health problems. For example, patients with inflammatory bowel disease, such as ulcerative colitis or enteritis that affects the lower bowel, should be very cautious about receiving radiation and are generally advised to have surgery instead. Attitudes toward incontinence, erectile dysfunction, and the potential need for additional therapy are other factors that come into play. For some men, the risk of surgical complications is too great, and therefore radiation becomes the best option.

Some research—including a 2016 analysis that pooled 19 studies involving a total of 118,830 men with low-, intermediate-, or high-risk prostate cancer—shows that surgically treated men have longer survival. Similarly, a 2021 review of data on 24,407 men with high-risk or very high-risk prostate cancer found that survival rates were better at five years of follow-up when the men were treated with surgery instead of radiation. But the evidence is not straightforward: a 2019 study, for instance, found no difference in survival among 10,439 men with unfavorable intermediate-risk prostate cancer who were treated with radical prostatectomy or radiation. Dr. Garnick cautions that the evidence so far also comes from retrospective studies that may not have fully

continued on page 69

Outcomes of prostate cancer surgery

Alenizi AM, Zorn KC, Bienz M, et al. Erectile Function Recovery After Robotic-Assisted Radical Prostatectomy (RARP): Long Term Exhaustive Analysis Across All Preoperative Potency Categories. *Canadian Journal of Urology* 2016;23(5):8451–56. PMID: 27705730.

Capogrosso P, Vertosick EA, Benfante NE, et al. Are We Improving Erectile Function Recovery After Radical Prostatectomy? Analysis of Patients Treated Over the Last Decade. *European Urology* 2019;75(2):221–28. PMID: 30237021.

Coughlin GD, Yaxley JW, Chambers SK, et al. Robot-Assisted Laparoscopic Prostatectomy Versus Open Radical Retropubic Prostatectomy: 24-Month Outcomes from a Randomized Controlled Study. *Lancet Oncology* 2018;19(8):1051–60. PMID: 30017351.

Favorito LA. Age and Body Mass Index: The Most Important Factors of Urinary and Erectile Function Recovery After Robotic Assisted Radical Prostatectomy. *International Brazilian Journal of Urology* 2019;45(4):653–54. PMID: 31397985.

Hoffman KE, Penson DF, Zhao Z, et al. Patient-Reported Outcomes Through 5 Years for Active Surveillance, Surgery, Brachytherapy, or External Beam Radiation With or Without Androgen Deprivation Therapy for Localized Prostate Cancer. *JAMA* 2020;323(2):149–63. PMID: 31935027.

Lee JK, Assel M, Thong AE, et al. Unexpected Long-Term Improvements in Urinary and Erectile Function in a Large Cohort of Men with Self-Reported Outcomes Following Radical Prostatectomy. *European Urology* 2015;68(5):899–905. PMID: 26293181.

Trieu D, Ju IE, Chang SB, et al. Surgeon Case Volume and Continence Recovery Following Radical Prostatectomy: A Systematic Review. *ANZ Journal of Surgery* 2021;91(4):521–29. PMID: 33319438.

PubMed See page 120.

<table>
<tr><th colspan="6">Table 5. Forms of radiation therapy</th></tr>
<tr><th>Treatment</th><th>Ideal candidates</th><th>Treatment time and recovery</th><th>Side effects</th><th>Advantages</th><th>Disadvantages</th></tr>
<tr><td>Standard external beam radiation techniques: three-dimensional conformal radiation therapy (3D-CRT) and intensity-modulated radiation therapy (IMRT)</td><td rowspan="4">Older patients or those with multiple medical conditions; patients whose cancer has spread outside the prostate capsule; men who have had a transurethral resection of the prostate (TURP).</td><td rowspan="2">35 to 45 treatments (five times a week for seven to nine weeks); each treatment takes about 15 minutes.</td><td rowspan="4">Bowel problems (diarrhea, blood in stool, rectal leakage, rectal pain), frequent urination, blood in the urine, urinary incontinence (increases over time), impotence (develops slowly), fatigue.</td><td>Both 3D-CRT and IMRT are very well-understood therapies with well-documented outcomes.
IMRT may, in theory, allow more accurate targeting of the tumor than 3D-CRT so that there's less damage to surrounding healthy tissue. The intensity of each of the beams can be adjusted.</td><td>Length of treatment makes it inconvenient, especially for men living far away from a treatment facility or those who travel frequently.
In rare cases, the radiation may miss part of the tumor if the beam is too narrowly focused.</td></tr>
<tr><td>Proton beam therapy</td><td>May be able to deliver more radiation to the prostate and less to surrounding tissues, causing less damage to nearby structures; protons release their energy after traveling a certain distance, limiting damage to the tissue they pass through.</td><td>Available at a limited number of sites in the United States.
Might not be covered by insurance.
More research is needed to determine whether it reduces side effects.</td></tr>
<tr><td>Stereotactic body radiation therapy (e.g., CyberKnife, Gamma Knife)</td><td>Usually five outpatient treatments, each lasting 60 to 90 minutes. May require fewer treatments if combined with another form of radiation.</td><td>Corrects for small movements and changes in the prostate during the course of treatment.
Shorter treatment time is important for some men.</td><td>Limited availability.
Short-term data suggest equal efficacy to other forms of radiation therapy.</td></tr>
<tr><td>Hypofractionated radiation therapy</td><td>Five outpatient treatments, which can be done in a single week or spread out over five weeks.</td><td>The shorter treatment time is important for some men, especially those living in areas without easy access to radiation facilities.</td><td>Limited data available on outcomes after five years.</td></tr>
<tr><td>Permanent seed implants (brachytherapy)</td><td>Men with early-stage cancer and prostate volume of less than 60 ml.</td><td>Half-day to full-day outpatient procedure with anesthesia.</td><td rowspan="2">Impotence and urinary and bowel problems.
Pain and rectal irritation usually resolve in about a month.</td><td rowspan="2">Radiation is concentrated in the prostate, potentially sparing the urethra, bladder, rectum, and nerves.
Can be used with external beam radiation in high-risk patients.</td><td>Small risk that unlinked seeds will migrate or be passed in the urine. Rarely, seeds enter the bloodstream and travel to the lungs or other parts of the body.
May cause severe urinary toxicity, which may last a long time.</td></tr>
<tr><td>High-dose-rate brachytherapy</td><td>Intermediate- and high-risk patients.</td><td>Usually three treatments over a few days; treatments last about 15 minutes.</td><td>Limited availability.
Needles remain in place until after the final treatment.
Requires a hospital stay.</td></tr>
</table>

Table 6. Percentage of patients with side effects three years after radiation

Type of radiation therapy	Percentage of men with urinary incontinence	Percentage of men with erectile dysfunction
High-dose-rate brachytherapy	7%	72%
Low-dose-rate brachytherapy	5.4%	36%
External beam radiation therapy (generally 3D-CRT, IMRT, and stereotactic)	2.7% (4% after six years)	68% (73% after six years)

Sources: Donovan JL, Hamdy FC, Lane JA, et al. Patient-reported Outcomes After Monitoring, Surgery, or Radiotherapy for Prostate Cancer. *New England Journal of Medicine* 2016;375(15):1425–37. PMID: 27626365.

Smith DP, King MT, Egger S, et al. Quality of Life Three Years After Diagnosis of Localized Prostate Cancer: Population Based Cohort Study. *BMJ* 2009;339:b4817. PMID: 19945997.

continued from page 67

considered the impact of age and health problems other than the cancer (see "Keeping statistics in perspective," page 70). Men who undergo radiation tend to be older with additional health problems, while those who undergo surgery tend to be younger and fitter with fewer pretreatment urinary and sexual problems and a better overall prognosis.

The most common side effects of radiation therapy are bowel problems (such as diarrhea, blood in the stool, and rectal pain) and urinary difficulties, as well as erectile dysfunction, which generally develops later on (see Table 6, above). Several of these problems may worsen with time. And studies have also shown a small but definite increased incidence of rectal cancer after radiation therapy. Researchers are investigating ways to reduce these side effects by modifying treatments. (For references, see "Radiation vs. surgery," at right.)

Surgery combined with radiation

Giving radiation after surgery is generally recommended when a man's cancer has begun growing beyond the prostate capsule or into other tissues nearby (see "Radiation treatment after prostatectomy," page 75). Alternatively, men in this high-risk group may be given a combination of radiation and hormonal therapy, without surgery. The optimal treatment approach is widely debated. A 2018 study provided the first evidence that long-term prostate cancer–specific survival rates are better with surgery plus radiation. During the study, researchers combed through medical claims data of 13,856 men ages 65 or older who were diagnosed with locally advanced prostate cancer between 1992 and 2009. Of them, 3,272 were treated with radiation and hormonal therapy, and 848 had surgery followed by radiation. After a follow-up period averaging 10 years, 89% of the men in the surgery-plus-radiation group had avoided death from prostate cancer, compared with 74.2% of men in the radiation-plus-hormonal-therapy group. Follow-up prospective research is needed to confirm the findings. (For reference, see "Surgery combined with radiation," at right.)

Radiation vs. surgery

Chierigo F, Wenzel M, Würnschimmel C, et al. Survival After Radical Prostatectomy Versus Radiation Therapy in High-Risk and Very High-Risk Prostate Cancer. *Journal of Urology* 2022;207(2):375–84. PMID: 34555930.

Eisemann N, Nolte S, Schnoor M, et al. The ProCaSP Study: Quality of Life Outcomes of Prostate Cancer Patients After Radiotherapy or Radical Prostatectomy in a Cohort Study. *BMC Urology* 2015;15:28. PMID: 25885890.

Huang H, Muscatelli S, Naslund M, et al. Evaluation of Cancer Specific Mortality with Surgery Versus Radiation as Primary Therapy for Localized High Grade Prostate Cancer in Men Younger than 60 Years. *Journal of Urology* 2019;201(1):120–28. PMID: 30059685.

Marsh S, Walters RW, Silberstein PT. Survival Outcomes of Radical Prostatectomy Versus Radiotherapy in Intermediate-Risk Prostate Cancer: A NCDB Study. *Clinical Genitourinary Cancer* 2018;16(1):e39–46. PMID: 28869138.

Resnick MJ, Koyama T, Fan KH, et al. Long-Term Functional Outcomes After Treatment for Localized Prostate Cancer. *New England Journal of Medicine* 2013;368(5):436–45. PMID: 23363497.

Sebastian NT, McElroy JP, Martin DD, et al. Survival After Radiotherapy vs. Radical Prostatectomy for Unfavorable Intermediate-Risk Prostate Cancer. *Urologic Oncology* 2019;37(11):813.e11–19. PMID: 31109836.

Tilki D, Chen MH, Wu J, et al. Surgery vs Radiotherapy in the Management of Biopsy Gleason Score 9–10 Prostate Cancer and the Risk of Mortality. *JAMA Oncology* 2019;5(2):213–20. PMID: 30452521.

Wallis CJ, Saskin R, Choo R, et al. Surgery Versus Radiotherapy for Clinically-Localized Prostate Cancer: A Systematic Review and Meta-Analysis. *European Urology* 2016;70(1):21–30. PMID: 26700655.

Surgery combined with radiation

Jang TL, Patel N, Faiena I, et al. Comparative Effectiveness of Radical Prostatectomy with Adjuvant Radiotherapy Versus Radiotherapy Plus Androgen Deprivation Therapy for Men with Advanced Prostate Cancer. *Cancer* 2018;124(20):4010–22. PMID: 30252932.

PubMed See page 120.

External beam radiation

During external beam radiation therapy (see Figure 8, below), rays of high-energy radiation are aimed directly at portions of the prostate gland that contain the tumor (and sometimes at nearby lymph nodes). External beam radiation effectively destroys cancer cells, but it can also damage adjoining healthy tissue. To limit the collateral damage, a specialist determines the exact location of the tumor using a CT scanner. This technology relays images to a computer that constructs a detailed three-dimensional map of the prostate and seminal vesicles. The map allows the radiation therapist to precisely target the cancerous tissue while avoiding the healthy tissue nearby. The therapist places the patient on the table in exactly the right position, checks the computer settings, and finally activates the device that delivers the radiation. (For general references on this approach, see "External beam radiation therapy," below left.)

Several types of external beam radiation therapy are used:

Three-dimensional conformal radiation therapy (3D-CRT) was once the standard form of outpatient radiation therapy. It involves taking three-dimensional pictures of the prostate and surrounding structures before treatment to pinpoint their locations. Using computer software, specialists determine the angles at which the beams of radiation should enter the tissue. In this way, the radiation field conforms to the shape of the treatment area and helps keep radiation away from the bladder and rectum. Typically 35 to 45 treatments are required—five times a week for seven to nine weeks, with each treatment taking about 15 minutes.

Keeping statistics in perspective

The research on outcomes after surgery, radiation, and other types of prostate cancer treatments has focused mainly on men diagnosed on the basis of symptoms. There is still no proof that any of these interventions prevent death or even extend lives in men whose prostate cancers were diagnosed on the basis of screening with PSA tests and who had no symptoms.

External beam radiation therapy

Goy BW, Burchette R, Soper MS, et al. Ten-Year Treatment Outcomes of Radical Prostatectomy Vs External Beam Radiation Therapy Vs Brachytherapy for 1503 Patients with Intermediate-Risk Prostate Cancer. *Urology* 2020;136:180–89. PMID: 31704459.

Greco C, Vazirani AA, Pares O, et al. The Evolving Role of External Beam Radiotherapy in Localized Prostate Cancer. *Seminars in Oncology* 2019;46(3):246–53. PMID: 31492437.

Figure 8. External beam radiation therapy

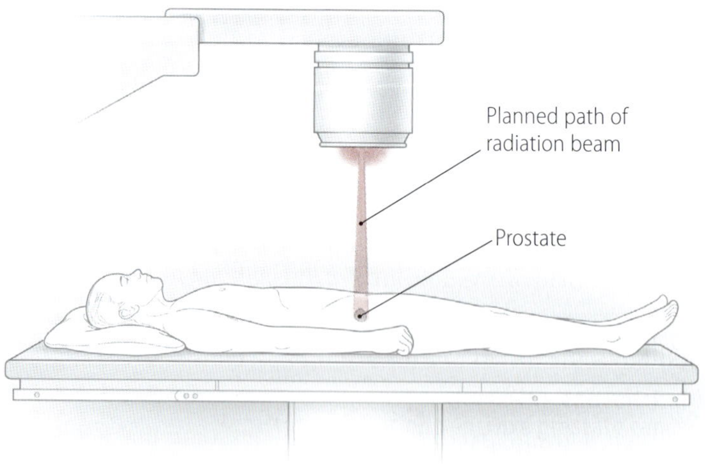

During external beam radiation for prostate cancer, a patient will typically wear a gown or sweat pants that can easily be removed so that the area to be treated can be aligned with a ray of light that matches the path of the radiation. The radiation beam itself is not visible. Marks on the skin or metallic gold implants (called gold fiducials) in the prostate help pinpoint the gland's location. The patient may also lie in a custom-made body "cast" to immobilize the pelvis.

Intensity-modulated radiation therapy (IMRT) is a form of 3D-CRT that allows doctors to change the intensity of the radiation within each of the radiation beams—increasing radiation to the prostate while reducing radiation to normal tissues. Because treatment conforms so tightly to the prostate, the gland's exact location must be determined at the start of each treatment. This is now the most commonly used form of radiation therapy in the United States. Research published in 2019 showed that using IMRT to treat the pelvic lymph nodes in men with high-grade prostate cancer resulted in no bowel or bladder side effects at three years. But the authors cautioned that more research is needed to confirm the anti-cancer effectiveness of that broader treatment. (For references, see "Intensity-modulated radiation therapy," at right.) As with 3D-CRT, 35 to 45 treatments are typically used—five times a week for seven to nine weeks, with each treatment taking about 15 minutes.

Proton beam therapy exhibits the same precision as IMRT, but it uses protons (subatomic particles with a positive electrical charge) instead of photons (light particles), which are used in conventional radiation. During proton beam therapy, radiation is released in a very narrow band, thus theoretically minimizing damage to surrounding tissue. A 2019 study with 307 men who were previously treated with surgery for prostate cancer showed that while proton beam therapy resulted in lower off-target doses to the bladder and rectum than IMRT, there was no difference between the two therapies with respect to bowel or bladder side effects at five years. Other studies have reached conflicting conclusions. A 2016 review concluded that proton beam therapy offers no significant advantage over IMRT for prostate cancer treatment, but a 2021 study found it was associated with longer overall survival. Proton beam therapy is more expensive, so few private insurers will cover it. Dr. Garnick says that ideally, all men receiving proton beam therapy would be enrolled in a clinical trial so that the risks and benefits of the therapy would be discovered in a well-designed study. At this time, proton beam therapy is available at only a few centers because it requires a cyclotron (a type of particle accelerator that is prohibitively expensive for many hospitals) to deliver the radiation. (For references, see "Proton beam therapy," at right.)

Stereotactic body radiation therapy (SBRT) uses image guidance and computer-controlled robotics to deliver multiple beams of radiation to the tumor from almost any direction. Several devices are available to deliver this form of radiation, so patients may also hear this method referred to as the CyberKnife, the Gamma Knife, TomoTherapy, or other brand names. While planning treatment, the radiologist implants tiny gold pellets called fiducials in the prostate gland to make it more visible for treatment purposes. The computer system tracks the tumor's position, detects prostate movement, and automatically adjusts the delivery of radiation, if necessary, to account for any change. SBRT is gaining in popularity because of its convenience (the method is faster than other forms of radiation, typically five high-dose sessions over one to two weeks) and potentially lower costs. Several recent review studies have shown that the method is safe and that it delays disease progression in patients with prostate cancer. A 2018 study found no difference in urinary, bowel, or erectile problems among men younger than 65 who were treated for prostate cancer with either SBRT or IMRT between 2008 and 2015, though SBRT was delivered at a lower cost. In 2020,

Intensity-modulated radiation therapy

Fischer-Valuck BW, Rao YJ, Michalski JM. Intensity-Modulated Radiotherapy for Prostate Cancer. *Translational Andrology and Urology* 2018;7(3):297–307. PMID: 30050791.

Parry M, Sujenthiran A, Cowling TE, et al. Treatment-Related Toxicity Using Prostate-Only Versus Prostate and Pelvic Lymph Node Intensity-Modulated Radiation Therapy: A National Population-Based Study. *Journal of Clinical Oncology* 2019;37(21):1828–35. PMID: 31163009.

Proton beam therapy

Liu Y, Patel SA, Jani AB, et al. Overall Survival After Treatment of Localized Prostate Cancer with Proton Beam Therapy, External-Beam Photon Therapy, or Brachytherapy. *Clinical Genitourinary Cancer* 2021;19(3):255–66.e7. PMID: 32972877.

Santos PMG, Barsky AR, Hwang TW, et al. Comparative Toxicity Outcomes of Proton-Beam Therapy Versus Intensity-Modulated Radiotherapy for Prostate Cancer in the Postoperative Setting. *Cancer* 2019;125(23):4278–93. PMID: 31503338.

Takagi M, Demizu Y, Fujii O, et al. Proton Therapy for Localized Prostate Cancer: Long-Term Results from a Single-Center Experience. *International Journal of Radiation Oncology, Biology, Physics* 2021;109(4):964–74. PMID: 33186616.

Yamoah K, Johnstone PA. Proton Beam Therapy: Clinical Utility and Current Status in Prostate Cancer. *OncoTargets and Therapy* 2016;9:5721–27. PMID: 27695349.

PubMed See page 120.

researchers published evidence that SBRT can also be safe and effective for men with oligometastatic prostate cancer (cancer that has spread to five or fewer different sites in the body, as detected by imaging). During the study, 54 men were randomized to either SBRT directed at cancer sites outside the prostate or to an observation group that received no treatment. After six months, the cancer had progressed in just 19% of the men in the radiation-treated group, compared with 61% of men in the observation group. Then in 2021, researchers published a study demonstrating that SBRT was effective in 344 men with high-risk cancer that was still localized to the prostate. After four years of follow-up, 81.7% of the men had avoided biochemical recurrence, and 89.1% of them were free of metastases. (For references, see "Stereotactic body radiation therapy," at left.)

Hypofractionated radiation therapy divides (fractionates) the total dose of radiation into larger doses that are given in fewer sessions than standard radiation therapy—typically, a total of five treatments over the course of one to five weeks. A 2019 review of 10 studies that compared hypofractionated and conventionally fractionated radiation therapy given to 8,278 men with early-stage prostate cancer found no differences in toxicity or survival after six years of follow-up. Clinical guidelines published jointly in 2018 by the American Society for Radiation Oncology, the American Society of Clinical Oncology, and the AUA concluded that despite limited follow-up beyond five years, the accumulated evidence so far warrants the use of hypofractionated therapy for men who would prefer it. The evidence is strongest for men with low- to intermediate-risk prostate cancer, given that most of the men treated in randomized controlled clinical trials fell into these categories. Still, men with high-risk cancer were also fairly well represented in the trials, and the position of the expert guidelines is that hypofractionated radiation therapy can be offered to men in all risk categories after a discussion with a doctor about the risks and benefits. The primary benefit of hypofractionated radiation is convenience, particularly for men who have to travel long distances for treatment. Some institutions will even provide housing for men while their treatment is under way. The main disadvantage is a shortage of information on long-term safety and efficacy. The criteria for selecting suitable candidates for hypofractionation vary by institution, and treatment protocols are continuing to evolve as researchers refine the optimal fractionations. (For references, see "Hypofractionated radiation therapy," at left.)

For most of these types of external beam radiation, certain advanced imaging techniques can assist the radiologist:

- Targeted delineation uses imaging technology to pinpoint radiation therapy. MRI scans can be used to locate tumors and plan where radiation should be targeted for maximum effect. Currently, MRI scans require the use of an endorectal coil inserted into the rectum, but a more powerful scanner (3-Tesla) allows MRI imaging of the gland without the coil.
- Positron emission tomography (PET), which does not require an endorectal coil, can produce an image of the gland and the location of tumors so that treatment can zero in on the cancer and spare surrounding tissue. PET scans use radioactive trac-

Stereotactic body radiation therapy

Connor MJ, Smith A, Miah S, et al. Targeting Oligometastasis with Stereotactic Ablative Radiation Therapy or Surgery in Metastatic Hormone-Sensitive Prostate Cancer: A Systematic Review of Clinical Trials. *European Urology Oncology* 2020;3(5):582–93. PMID: 32891600.

Malouff TD, Stross WC, Seneviratne DS, et al. Current Use of Stereotactic Body Radiation for Low and Intermediate Risk Prostate Cancer: A National Cancer Database Analysis. *Prostate Cancer and Prostatic Diseases* 2020;23(2):349–55. PMID: 31780782.

Pan HY, Jiang J, Hoffman KE, et al. Comparative Toxicities and Cost of Intensity-Modulated Radiotherapy, Proton Radiation, and Stereotactic Body Radiotherapy Among Younger Men with Prostate Cancer. *Journal of Clinical Oncology* 2018;36(18):1823–30. PMID: 29561693.

Philips R, Shi WY, Deek M, et al. Outcomes of Observation vs Stereotactic Ablative Radiation for Oligometastatic Prostate Cancer: The ORIOLE Phase 2 Randomized Clinical Trial. *JAMA Oncology* 2020;6(5):650–59. PMID: 32215577.

Van Dams R, Jiang NY, Fuller DB, et al. Stereotactic Body Radiotherapy for High-Risk Localized Carcinoma of the Prostate (SHARP) Consortium: Analysis of 344 Prospectively Treated Patients. *International Journal of Radiation Oncology, Biology, Physics* 2021;110(3):731–37. PMID: 33493615.

Hypofractionated radiation therapy

Hickey BE, James ML, Daly T, et al. Hypofractionation for Clinically Localized Prostate Cancer. *Cochrane Database of Systematic Reviews* 2019;9:CD011462. PMID: 31476800.

Morgan SC, Hoffman K, Loblaw DA, et al. Hypofractionated Radiation Therapy for Localized Prostate Cancer: An ASTRO, ASCO, and AUA Evidence-Based Guideline. *Journal of Clinical Oncology* 2018;36(34):3411–30. PMID: 30307776.

PubMed See page 120.

ers injected into the body that accumulate preferentially in cancer cells. Then, when the patient is placed under a PET scanner, the tracer signals the tumor's location. Newer tracers approved by the FDA bind specifically to the PSMA protein in the prostate cancer cell membrane (see "FDA approves the first PSMA-targeted PET imaging tracers," page 6). These tracers are also driving the development of new PSMA-targeted therapies that kill off metastatic cells in the body before they have a chance to form new tumors (see "A new treatment for advanced prostate cancer lengthens survival in clinical trials," page 6).

Brachytherapy

Rather than delivering radiation from an external source, brachytherapy delivers radiation from a source placed inside the body. *Brachy-* is Greek for "short," so brachytherapy refers to the radiation source being a short distance from the cancer. Sometimes brachytherapy is called internal radiation therapy or interstitial radiation therapy. The most common form of brachytherapy is permanent brachytherapy. Other names for it are low-dose-rate brachytherapy or seed implantation. This form of brachytherapy involves placing 50 to 150 radioactive pellets, or "seeds," in or near the prostate tumor (see Figure 9, below). The number of seeds depends on the size of the gland.

After the patient receives either general or spinal anesthesia, the doctor places an ultrasound probe in the man's rectum and a catheter in his bladder. Viewing a computerized map of the prostate, the doctor guides the placement of the seeds, using a

Figure 9. Permanent brachytherapy (seed implantation)

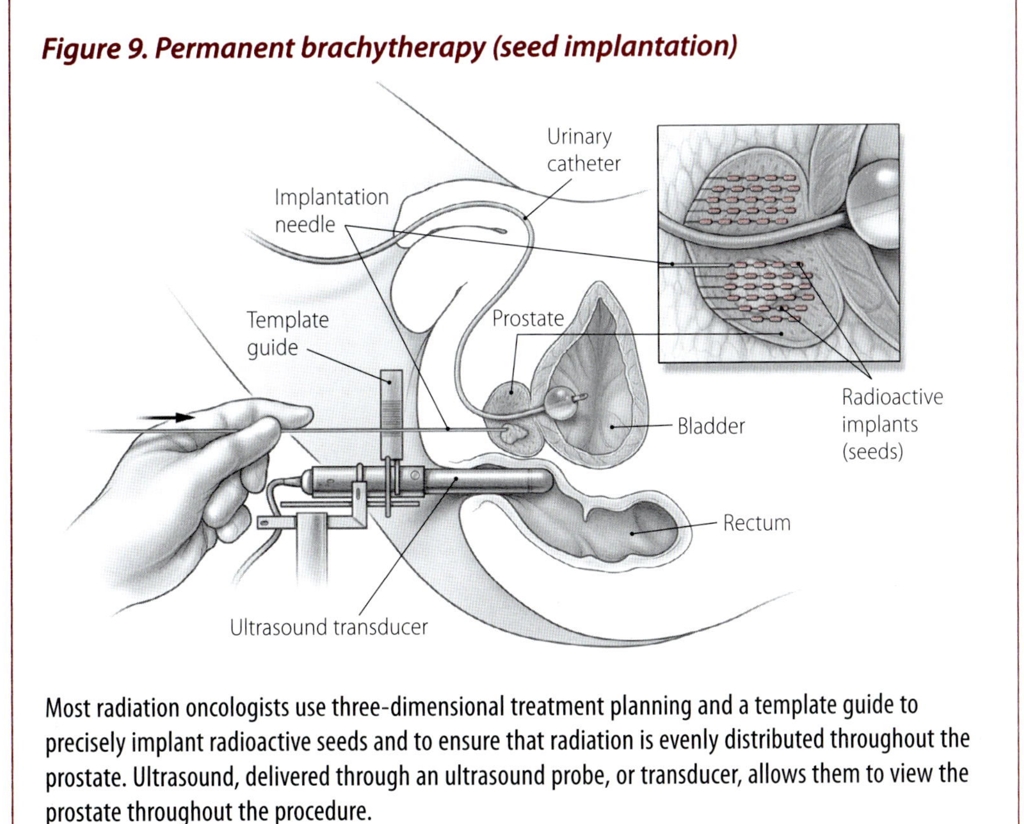

Most radiation oncologists use three-dimensional treatment planning and a template guide to precisely implant radioactive seeds and to ensure that radiation is evenly distributed throughout the prostate. Ultrasound, delivered through an ultrasound probe, or transducer, allows them to view the prostate throughout the procedure.

template and a needle to insert them through the perineum. Doctors leave the seeds, which are smaller than grains of rice, in place permanently. Over time, the seeds emit less and less radiation until they become nonradioactive. Depending on the type of seeds, the loss of radioactivity may take three months to a year.

One advantage of permanent brachytherapy is that it's usually an outpatient procedure. Most men go home as soon as the anesthesia wears off. If you have permanent brachytherapy, you will need to abstain from sex for about two weeks and then use a condom for several weeks to protect your partner from radiation exposure. In addition, the ejaculate may be bloody and low in volume at first.

However, brachytherapy may cause severe urinary tract side effects, such as bleeding, incontinence, and the urgent and frequent need to urinate. Although this is rare, the problem can last a long time—even after the seeds are no longer radioactive—because of damage done by the initial radiation. Dr. Garnick rarely, if ever, recommends brachytherapy as a first-line treatment for patients with localized prostate cancer. According to his observations, brachytherapy rates appear to be falling, given the potential for life-changing urinary consequences. However, he will consider salvage radiation together with brachytherapy if cancer recurs within the prostate gland (see "Radiation treatment after prostatectomy," page 75).

In very rare instances, a doctor may suggest a different type of brachytherapy called high-dose-rate brachytherapy, in which the seeds are temporarily placed and then removed several days later. As with permanent brachytherapy, the radioactive material is inserted into the prostate. But given the high intensity of the material, it cannot be left in the body for long. After a set period of time, a remote-controlled machine pulls the material out. The process is repeated over multiple days.

Focal therapy

Instead of removing the whole prostate, focal therapy treats only the part of the prostate where the cancer is located. Focal therapy has been likened to a lumpectomy done for breast cancer, targeting only the cancerous mass while sparing the rest of the breast. In the same way, focal therapy, which is still experimental in the United States, destroys the tumor while sparing the surrounding tissue. The hope is that this approach will not only remove the cancer, but also minimize side effects such as erectile dysfunction and urinary incontinence, which are commonly seen with prostate cancer treatment.

The evidence on focal therapy so far gives reason to be cautiously optimistic about the strategy. Focal therapy limits urinary incontinence and erectile dysfunction; in addition, biopsies after focal therapy show that the approach can eliminate clinically significant cancer. Studies have shown that most men who receive focal therapy for low- and intermediate-risk tumors remain free of urinary incontinence, sexual problems, and subsequent increases in their PSA levels for up to a year, and that during that time, fewer than one in 10 has a recurrence of his cancer. In a 2020 study, almost half of the 309 men who were given focal therapy for low- to intermediate-risk prostate cancer had no recurrence in five years. Furthermore, 98% of the cancers had not

continued on page 76

Radiation treatment after prostatectomy

Radiation can be first-line therapy for prostate cancer, but it is also used after radical prostatectomy (surgical removal of the prostate). Postsurgical radiation can take either of two forms:

- Adjuvant radiation is radiation therapy given soon after surgery when there is a high likelihood of residual cancer.
- Salvage radiation is radiation therapy given if radical prostatectomy hasn't fully worked—that is, the cancer has come back or PSA levels have started to rise (a condition called biochemical recurrence).

In 2013, the American Urological Association (AUA) and the American Society for Radiation Oncology (ASTRO) issued guidelines for both adjuvant and salvage radiation. The guidelines say that after prostatectomy, patients with pathological findings that suggest cancer is still present (as indicated by traces of cancer in the surgical margins surrounding the area where the prostate used to be) or evidence of cancer in tissues next to the prostate should be informed that adjuvant radiation therapy will reduce the risk of local recurrence and clinical progression, but that the effects on the potential for spread (metastasis) and survival are less clear. The AUA/ASTRO guidelines also state that patients with rising PSA levels after radical prostatectomy should be offered salvage radiation even without evidence of distant metastatic disease, and be told that radiation is likely to be most effective when PSA levels are low.

Adjuvant therapy rates are declining among men who have surgery for cancer with high-risk characteristics, and fewer than 20% of such patients opt for the additional radiation, given concerns about overtreatment, impotence, erectile dysfunction, and other side effects. The rest opt for observation and then salvage radiation if PSA levels start to rise. Results from two clinical trials published in 2020 suggested that radiation can be safely delayed until there is clear evidence of the cancer's return. After an average of five years, biochemical recurrence and prostate cancer–specific survival rates were similar regardless of whether men had received adjuvant radiation, and the radiation-treated men reported greater side effects, including urinary incontinence. Yet newer results from a 2021 paper suggest that adjuvant radiation may be a better option than early salvage radiation for men with Gleason scores of 8 to 10 that are already breaking through the prostate capsule. After a follow-up of nearly nine years, men who opted for adjuvant radiation had a significantly lower risk of death from all causes in addition to prostate cancer.

The AUA/ASTRO guidelines do not set a strict standard of care. Whether a patient should have adjuvant or salvage radiation needs to be decided on a case-by-case basis that factors in a man's overall health and outlook. New tests that look for biomarkers of aggressive cancer behavior and a tendency toward metastasis can help with treatment decisions (see "Biomarkers and genetic testing," page 97). However, in more recent amendments, the AUA/ASTRO guidelines stated that the present level of evidence is insufficient for these tools to predict the efficacy of either adjuvant or salvage radiation after surgery.

An important factor that predicts the likelihood of cancer returning is the Gleason score of cells in the surgical margins. Among men who have cancer cells in the margins after surgery, only half experience a recurrence of the cancer, and those who do generally had margin cells with higher Gleason scores. For that reason, Dr. Garnick recommends adjuvant radiation after radical prostatectomy if the surgical margins contain any Gleason pattern 4 or 5 cells.

Sources: Braide K, Kindblom J, Lindencrona U, et al. Salvage Radiation Therapy in Prostate Cancer: Relationship Between Rectal Dose and Long-Term, Self-Reported Rectal Bleeding. *Clinical and Translational Oncology* 2021;23(2):397–404. PMID: 32621207.

Chapin BF, Nguyen JN, Achim MF, et al. Positive Margin Length and Highest Gleason Grade of Tumor at the Margin Predict for Biochemical Recurrence After Radical Prostatectomy in Patients with Organ-Confined Prostate Cancer. *Prostate Cancer and Prostatic Diseases* 2018;21(2):221–27. PMID: 29230008.

Hackman G, Taari K, Tammela TL, et al. Randomised Trial of Adjuvant Radiotherapy Following Radical Prostatectomy Versus Radical Prostatectomy Alone in Prostate Cancer Patients with Positive Margins or Extracapsular Extension. *European Urology* 2019;76(5):586–95. PMID: 31375279.

Hwang WL, Tendulkar RD, Niemierko A, et al. Comparison Between Adjuvant and Early-Salvage Postprostatectomy Radiotherapy for Prostate Cancer with Adverse Pathological Features. *JAMA Oncology* 2018;4(5):e175320. PMID: 29372236.

Parker CC, Clarke NW, Cook AD, et al. Timing of Radiotherapy After Radical Prostatectomy (RADICALS-RT): A Randomized, Controlled Phase 3 Trial. *Lancet* 2020;396(10260):1413–21. PMID: 33002429.

Pisansky TM, Thompson IM, Valicenti RK, et al: Adjuvant and Salvage Radiotherapy After Prostatectomy: ASTRO/AUA Guideline Amendment 2018–2019. *Journal of Urology* 2019;202(3):533–38. PMID: 31042111.

Sargos P, Chabaoud S, Latorzeff I, et al. Adjuvant Radiotherapy vs Early Salvage Radiotherapy Plus Short-Term Androgen Deprivation Therapy in Men with Localized Prostate Cancer After Radical Prostatectomy (GETUG-AFU17): A Randomized, Phase 3 Trial. *Lancet Oncology* 2020;21(10):1341–52. PMID: 33002438.

Tendulkar RD, Agrawal S, Gao T, et al. Contemporary Update of a Multi-Institutional Predictive Nomogram for Salvage Radiotherapy After Radical Prostatectomy. *Journal of Clinical Oncology* 2016;34(30):3648–54. PMID: 27528718.

Tilki D, Chen MH, Wu J, et al. Adjuvant vs Early Salvage Radiation Therapy for Men at High Risk for Recurrence Following Radical Prostatectomy for Prostate Cancer and the Risk of Death. *Journal of Clinical Oncology* 2021;39(20):2284–93. PMID: 34086480.

continued from page 74

spread to other parts of the body, and none of the men had died from prostate cancer. (For references, see "Focal therapy," at left.)

Since focal therapy does not treat the entire prostate, it's essential to pinpoint the "index lesion"—that is, the part of the tumor with the highest cancer grade. Thanks to dramatic improvements in imaging technologies, such as MRI, physicians can use a mapping biopsy (see Figure 10, page 77) to locate the index lesion and determine whether a cancer has spread to the seminal vesicles.

Focal therapy is best understood as an overall approach to treatment—one that can use any of several different technologies to get rid of the cancer. The techniques used most often are cryotherapy, which involves freezing tissue, and high-intensity focused ultrasound, a more powerful version of the harmless sound waves used to create diagnostic images of the prostate. A comparison of these and other techniques, published in 2021, could not point to one approach as being superior to the others. However, the authors concluded that despite data on long-term benefits, focal therapy could be an appealing option for men with intermediate-risk prostate cancer.

Cryotherapy. Cryotherapy, also called cryosurgery or cryoablation, kills cancer cells by freezing them. Used for focal therapy, it appears to work well when treating a small, newly diagnosed tumor. However, it is not recommended for treating multifocal cancer (cancer that appears in more than one spot within the prostate).

Complications from cryotherapy may be severe. They include rectal fistula (an abnormal opening in the skin near the anus that leads to the rectum); urinary stress incontinence; and—most often—erectile dysfunction, which affects 47% to 100% of men after treatment because there's no way to avoid freezing and destroying some nerves. There is also the chance that some cancer will be left behind. A 2020 study with 61 men who were treated with cryotherapy for intermediate-risk tumors on one side of the prostate found no further evidence of clinically significant cancer after 18 months. However, Dr. Garnick cautions that this is relatively short follow-up. He does not recommend cryotherapy as a first choice for treating multifocal prostate cancer, but says it could potentially be used in patients who have residual or recurring prostate cancer after being treated with radiation. If you do consider it, make sure the doctor has extensive experience with the technique.

High-intensity focused ultrasound (HIFU). This method of delivering ultrasound generates intense, precisely targeted heat to destroy cancer tissue. HIFU is available in Great Britain and a few other countries for localized prostate cancer. In the United States, the FDA gave HIFU a more limited approval in 2015. Clinical guidelines for treating localized prostate cancer published in 2019 by the AUA, the American Society for Radiation Oncology, and the Society of Urologic Oncology state that low- and intermediate-risk patients considering focal therapy should be informed that it is not a standard care option because there isn't enough research comparing HIFU and standard treatment. Still, a study published in 2020 showed that among 100 patients with low- to high-risk localized prostate cancer who had been treated with HIFU at a single institution, 91% avoided radical prostatectomy for two years, and none experi-

Focal therapy

Abreu AL, Peretsman S, Iwata A, et al. High Intensity Focused Ultrasound Hemigland Ablation for Prostate Cancer: Initial Outcomes of a United States Series. *Journal of Urology* 2020;204(4):741–47. PMID: 32898975.

Chuang R, Kinnard A, Kwan L, et al. Hemigland Cryoablation of Clinically Significant Prostate Cancer: Intermediate-Term Follow-up via Magnetic Resonance Imaging Guided Biopsy. *Journal of Urology* 2020;204(5):941–49. PMID: 32985924.

Fallara G, Capogrosso P, Maggio P, et al. Erectile Function After Focal Therapy for Localized Prostate Cancer: A Systematic Review. *International Journal of Impotence Research* 2021;33(4):418–27. PMID: 32999435.

Hübner N, Shariat SF, Remzi M. Focal Therapy of Prostate Cancer. *Current Opinion in Urology* 2018;28(6):550–54. PMID: 30239415.

Kayano PP, Klotz L. Current Evidence for Focal Therapy and Partial Gland Ablation for Organ-Confined Prostate Cancer: Systematic Review of Literature Published in the Last 2 Years. *Current Opinion in Urology* 2021;31(1):49–57. PMID: 33196540.

Sanda MG, Cadeddu JA, Kirkby E, et al. Clinically Localized Prostate Cancer: AUA/ASTRO/SUO Guideline. Part 1: Risk Stratification, Shared Decision Making, and Care Options. *Journal of Urology* 2018;199(3):683–90. PMID: 29203269.

Tourinho-Barbosa RR, Sanchez-Salas R, Claros OR, et al. Focal Therapy for Localized Prostate Cancer with Either High Intensity Focused Ultrasound or Cryoablation: A Single Institution Experience. *Journal of Urology* 2020;203(2):320–30. PMID: 31437121.

PubMed See page 120.

enced urinary incontinence. Moreover, in 73% of the men, the cancer did not progress over this two-year period.

Dr. Garnick was on an FDA panel charged with reviewing HIFU. He never recommends it as primary therapy, but adds that like cryotherapy, it may be considered for certain carefully selected men who have recurring or residual prostate cancer after radiation therapy.

Hormonal therapy (androgen deprivation therapy, or ADT)

Androgens, the family of male sex hormones that includes testosterone, function as a fuel for growth in normal development. However, in some men they can also drive the progression of prostate cancer. Hormonal therapy—also called androgen deprivation therapy (ADT)—treats prostate cancer by dramatically reducing levels of testosterone and other androgens. Hormonal therapy is a treatment option for men who

- have newly diagnosed cancer that has spread beyond the prostate gland (metastatic disease)
- have a rising PSA after initial treatment with surgery or radiation therapy, indicating a possible recurrence of cancer that may not be visible yet with standard imaging
- are frail and unable to tolerate surgery or radiation as their initial treatment.

In such cases, hormonal therapy is typically given by itself. But it can also be given in combination with other treatments, such as radiation and chemotherapy. In some cases, doctors prescribe it to boost the effectiveness of radiation therapy or to reduce the size of the tumor and prostate before brachytherapy (see "Combined hormonal therapy and radiation therapy," page 83).

Hormonal therapy uses drugs to lower androgen levels and slow prostate cancer (see Table 7, page 78). The older method of lowering male hormones—surgical removal of the testicles, the source of 90% of a man's testosterone—is rarely used today; hormonal therapy produces the same benefits without being permanent. If cancer continues to progress after hormonal therapy, it is referred to as castration-resistant prostate cancer; if it responds to hormonal therapy, it is called castration-sensitive.

In order for hormonal therapy to work, though, patients must take the prescribed medications as scheduled. Doctors often recommend injectable drugs—primarily those in a class known as luteinizing hormone–releasing hormone (LHRH) agonists (also called LHRH analogs, gonadotropin-releasing hormone [GnRH] agonists, or GnRH analogs). Two other classes of drugs, GnRH antagonists and anti-androgens, are also used.

Therapies that affect the pituitary gland

LHRH agonists stimulate the brain's pituitary gland—the gland whose hormones orchestrate the activity of other glands and hormones—resulting in a temporary surge

continued on page 79

Figure 10. Mapping biopsy

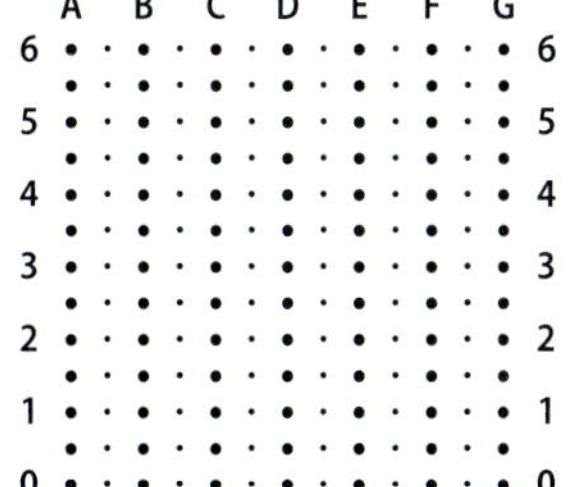

During a mapping biopsy, prostate tissue samples are taken every 5 millimeters, front to back and side to side. The radiologist places a grid over the perineum to aid the process. Each dot on the grid represents a hole through which a needle can be inserted. This allows doctors to map the location of tumors in three dimensions and determine if a patient might be a candidate for focal therapy.

Table 7. Hormonal therapy medications

Drug name	Side effects	Comments
LHRH agonists		
goserelin (Zoladex) histrelin (Vantas) leuprolide (Eligard, Lupron Depot) triptorelin (Trelstar)	Hot flashes, impotence, decreased libido, fatigue, weight gain, anemia, osteoporosis.	Injected or implanted.
GnRH antagonists		
degarelix (Firmagon)	Hot flashes, sleep disturbances, pain, dizziness, headache, nausea, fatigue; for degarelix, large welts at the injection site.	Given monthly via injection.
relugolix (Orgovyx)		Taken orally once a day.
Anti-androgens		
apalutamide (Erleada)	Fatigue, high blood pressure, rash, diarrhea, nausea, weight loss, joint pain, hot flashes, falls, decreased appetite, skeletal fractures, and swelling of extremities.	Taken orally. Approved for use in men with nmCRPC and mCSPC.
bicalutamide (Casodex)	Hot flashes, impotence, decreased libido, breast tenderness and swelling, nausea, diarrhea; rarely, liver failure.	Taken orally. Liver function should be checked periodically.
darolutamide (Nubeqa)	Fatigue, pain in extremities, and rash.	Taken orally twice daily with food. Approved for nmCRPC. Men should also take an LHRH agonist.
enzalutamide (Xtandi)	Fatigue, musculoskeletal pain, hot flashes, diarrhea, tissue swelling, respiratory infections, dizziness, difficulty sleeping, blood in urine, anxiety, high blood pressure. Seizures occur in about 1% of men.	Taken orally. Approved for mCRPC, nmCRPC, and mCSPC.
flutamide (Eulexin) nilutamide (Nilandron)	Hot flashes, impotence, decreased libido, breast tenderness and swelling, nausea, diarrhea; rarely, liver failure.	Taken orally. Liver function should be checked periodically.
Other		
abiraterone (Zytiga)	Joint swelling or discomfort, low levels of blood potassium, fluid retention in legs and feet, increased blood pressure, muscle aches, hot flashes, and urinary and gastrointestinal problems.	Used in combination with low-dose steroids. Approved as both first-line and second-line treatment for mCRPC.
estrogens	Blood clots and breast enlargement.	Once the main alternative to surgical removal of the testicles, these drugs have been largely replaced by LHRH agonists and anti-androgens. May be tried if other hormonal therapies don't work.
ketoconazole (Nizoral)	Dizziness, depression, headaches, loss of libido.	Used first for treating fungal infections, ketoconazole reduces testosterone levels quickly in men with advanced prostate cancer when other forms of hormonal therapy don't work.

Note: For abbreviations of tumor types, see "Prostate cancer terminology," page 38.

continued from page 77

in testosterone that generally lasts from three to four weeks. After that, this effect is reversed and testosterone levels decrease. During this initial period, symptoms such as bone pain may worsen, a situation known as a clinical flare. To counteract the testosterone surge during this period, LHRH agonists are often taken with other drugs called anti-androgens (see page 80) that prevent testosterone and its metabolite dihydrotestosterone from interacting with a protein in the prostate cancer cell called the androgen receptor. This two-pronged strategy, known as a combined hormone blockade, helps to reduce bone pain and produces more rapid declines in PSA than LHRH agonists given alone. Anti-androgens are taken orally and may also be prescribed to block the effect of additional testosterone secreted into the body by the adrenal glands (which produce about 5% to 10% of male hormones).

GnRH antagonists are another option for lowering testosterone levels by manipulating the pituitary gland. These drugs do not cause an initial testosterone surge. Degarelix (Firmagon),* which is given by injection once a month, was the first drug in this class. A 2016 review paper showed that for up to a year, degarelix and two LHRH agonists—goserelin (Zoladex) and leuprolide (Eligard, Lupron Depot)—had about the same PSA-lowering effect in patients with advanced prostate cancer, although the declines were at first more pronounced with degarelix. PSA was more likely to rise after degarelix treatment if a man had metastatic prostate cancer, or if his PSA level was 20 ng/ml or higher when he started taking the drug. The authors cautioned that the two drug classes still need to be compared in terms of how they affect survival. Clinical trials comparing the two drug classes are ongoing.

A 2020 review of 13 published studies showed that degarelix may be helpful for men who are no longer responding to LHRH agonists. Results from that review suggested that switching to degarelix after LHRH agonists fail can stabilize or reduce PSA levels in about 30% of patients within three months. However, the data were insufficient to determine how long this reduction lasts or whether it has a bearing on long-term outcomes for men with prostate cancer.

Concerns have arisen about the effects of both these types of drugs on cardiovascular health. In 2019, researchers published a study of 80 men with prostate cancer and cardiovascular disease who were treated with either an LHRH agonist or a GnRH antagonist for a year. Results showed that 3% of the men treated with the GnRH antagonist experienced new cardiovascular problems, compared with 20% of the LHRH agonist–treated men. That finding led to speculation that the GnRH antagonists are better for heart health. Yet highly anticipated findings published in 2021 failed to confirm this. The investigators compared 545 men randomized to a year's treatment with either the GnRH antagonist degarelix or the LHRH agonist leuprolide and could find no significant difference in heart-related outcomes between them. (For more information, see "Highly anticipated study of cardiovascular risk from different hormonal therapies ends in a draw," page 8.)

A second GnRH antagonist, called relugolix (Orgovyx),* was approved for advanced prostate cancer in late 2020. It is given in a convenient pill form (versus the monthly injection for degarelix). In a late-stage trial, it suppressed testosterone to opti-

**Editor's note:* Dr. Marc Garnick, editor in chief of the* Annual, *previously served as a consultant to Ferring Pharmaceuticals, the manufacturer of degarelix. He also served on a scientific board for Myovant, the manufacturer of relugolix, but has no current relationship with either company.*

mal levels within four days, and testosterone levels returned to normal within 90 days after men stopped taking the drug. Relugolix also appears to have fewer cardiovascular side effects than the LHRH agonists.

These and other side effects from hormonal therapies, including LHRH agonists and GnRH antagonists, are being studied in clinical trials. (For references, see "Degarelix and LHRH agonists," at left.)

Anti-androgens

Enzymes in the prostate convert testosterone into dihydrotestosterone (DHT), and it's DHT that stimulates the growth of prostate cells—and prostate cancer cells, if they're present. The goal of the anti-androgens is to keep DHT on the sidelines, idle and frustrated, by preventing it from binding to the androgen receptors on prostate cells. Several different drugs can do this. The traditional anti-androgens are bicalutamide (Casodex), flutamide (Eulexin), and nilutamide (Nilandron).

Newer anti-androgens include apalutamide (Erleada), darolutamide (Nubeqa), and enzalutamide (Xtandi). These drugs were all approved on the basis of their ability to delay the appearance of metastases in men with rising PSA levels (therefore increasing what's called metastasis-free survival) after initial prostate cancer treatment. The drugs have also been shown to delay the time to pain progression (worsening pain), bone problems, and the need for subsequent chemotherapy. They can be used in various settings. In some cases, doctors give an anti-androgen for a few weeks before treatment with an LHRH agonist, and in other cases, for the duration of LHRH treatment. Anti-androgens are generally not given together with GnRH agonists. They have a number of side effects. For example, enzalutamide causes seizures in a very small number of men (less than 1%; see "Side effects of hormonal therapy," page 81).

Enzalutamide. This drug was approved initially by the FDA in 2012 for men with metastatic castration-resistant prostate cancer (mCRPC; see "Prostate cancer terminology," page 38) who no longer respond to docetaxel (Taxotere), the main chemotherapy drug used for prostate cancer. That approval was subsequently extended to men who have not yet had chemotherapy after research showed the drug delayed the need for chemotherapy treatment by 17 months. Then, in 2018, enzalutamide was approved for *non*metastatic castration-resistant prostate cancer (nmCRPC) when a study published that year showed it prolonged metastasis-free survival for 14.7 months. In 2019, more findings showed the drug also delayed disease progression and extended survival in men with metastatic castration-*sensitive* prostate cancer (mCSPC). The drug was subsequently approved for that use as well.

Apalutamide. In 2018, the FDA approved apalutamide for nmCRPC after a study published that year showed that metastasis-free survival lasted two years longer in men taking the drug than it did in men who took a placebo. Then in 2019, the FDA extended apalutamide's approval to mCSPC, after a clinical trial with 525 men showed the drug delayed progression of the disease and also extended survival when it was given together with first-line hormonal therapy. A final analysis of this study, published in 2021, showed the drug also improved quality of life and delayed castration resistance.

Degarelix and LHRH agonists

Atchia KS, Walls CJD, Fleshner N, et al. Switching from a Gonadotropin-Releasing Hormone (GnRH) Agonist to a GnRH Antagonist in Prostate Cancer Patients: A Systematic Review and Meta-Analysis. *Canadian Urological Association Journal* 2020;14(2):36–41. PMID: 31348745.

Freedland SJ, Abrahamsson PA. Androgen Deprivation Therapy and Side Effects: Are GnRH Antagonists Safer? *Asian Journal of Andrology* 2021;23(1):3–10. PMID: 32655041.

Lopes RD, Higano CS, Slovin SF, et al. Cardiovascular Safety of Degarelix Versus Leuprolide in Patients with Prostate Cancer: The Primary Results of the PRONOUNCE Randomized Trial. *Circulation* 2021;144(16):1295–307. PMID: 34459214.

Margel D, Peer A, Ber Y. Cardiovascular Morbidity in a Randomized Trial Comparing GnRH Agonist and GnRH Antagonist Among Patients with Advanced Prostate Cancer and Preexisting Cardiovascular Disease. *Journal of Urology* 2019;202(6):1199–208. PMID: 31188734.

Motlagh RS, Abufaraj M, Mori K, et al. The Efficacy and Safety of Relugolix Compared with Degarelix in Advanced Prostate Cancer Patients: A Network Meta-Analysis of Randomized Trials. *European Urology and Oncology* 2021;Electronic publication ahead of print. PMID: 34301529.

Sciarra A, Fasulo A, Ciardi A, et al. A Meta-Analysis and Systematic Review of Randomized Controlled Trials with Degarelix Versus Gonadotropin-Releasing Hormone Agonists for Advanced Prostate Cancer. *Medicine (Baltimore)* 2016;95(27):e3845. PMID: 27399062.

PubMed See page 120.

Darolutamide. In 2019, the FDA approved darolutamide for nmCRPC after clinical trial results showed the drug extended metastasis-free survival for 40.4 months, compared with 18.4 months in men who took a placebo. The researchers continued studying the enrolled patients and reported in 2020 that the darolutamide-treated men also had modest improvements in overall survival: 83% of the men were still alive after three years, compared with 77% of placebo-treated men. (For references on all the drugs discussed in this section, see "Anti-androgens," at right.)

Abiraterone

Abiraterone (Zytiga) is another option for advanced prostate cancer. Approved by the FDA in 2011, abiraterone lowers testosterone levels by inhibiting an enzyme that is essential to the synthesis of the hormone. Indeed, it blocks the testosterone synthesis that occurs inside the prostate cancer cell itself. Abiraterone is given with prednisone, a powerful anti-inflammatory medication.

The FDA often initially approves drugs for a fairly narrow purpose, and abiraterone was first approved for use in men with who had already been treated with docetaxel. But like enzalutamide, it's since been approved for use before chemotherapy, and thus delays the need for treatments with more significant side effects.

In 2017, two major studies reported simultaneously that when given with other hormonal treatments to men with newly diagnosed aggressive prostate cancer, abiraterone reduced the odds that the men would die of their disease by up to 40% at 30 to 40 months of follow-up. That good news came after a 2015 study found that after being given abiraterone, men lived almost five months longer than patients who were given a control therapy. Importantly, abiraterone delayed the need for opiate pain medications by nearly a year, the investigators found.

Researchers also wondered if giving abiraterone and enzalutamide in any particular sequence might work better, but research indicates that it does not. A 2020 review of the published literature concluded that giving abiraterone before enzalutamide leads to a slower progression of the disease and longer-lasting control of PSA levels, but without any difference in survival.

There are also downsides. In the study that led to expanded use of abiraterone, about 10% of the patients dropped out because of the side effects. Moreover, nearly all patients eventually develop resistance to abiraterone as well as enzalutamide, and those who have a genetic mutation called AR-V7 affecting the testosterone receptor won't respond to either drug at all. (For references, see "Abiraterone and enzalutamide," page 82.)

Side effects of hormonal therapy

Not surprisingly, hormonal therapy can have a wide range of side effects, because it involves blocking a major hormone. Sexual dysfunction is most common, and hot flashes are not unusual. Some patients lose muscle mass or experience breast enlargement on these drugs. In addition, the anti-androgens have been linked to liver failure, so patients who take them should have routine tests of liver function. Hormonal therapy may also increase the risk of heart disease, so it is important to monitor risk

Anti-androgens

Armstrong AJ, Szmulewitz R, Petrylak DP, et al. ARCHES: A Randomized, Phase III Study of Androgen Deprivation Therapy with Enzalutamide or Placebo in Men with Metastatic Hormone-Sensitive Prostate Cancer. *Journal of Clinical Oncology* 2019;37(32):2974–86. PMID: 31329516.

Chi KN, Agarwal N, Bjartell, et al. Apalutamide for Metastatic, Castration-Sensitive Prostate Cancer. *New England Journal of Medicine* 2019;381(1):13–24. PMID: 31150574.

Chi KN, Chowdhury S, Bjartell A, et al. Apalutamide in Patients with Metastatic Castration-Sensitive Prostate Cancer: Final Survival Analysis of the Randomized, Double-Blind, Phase III TITAN study. *Journal of Clinical Oncology* 2021;39(20):2294–303. PMID: 33914595.

Davis ID, Martin AJ, Stockler MR, et al. Enzalutamide with Standard First-Line Therapy in Metastatic Prostate Cancer. *New England Journal of Medicine* 2019;381(2):121–31. PMID: 31157964.

Fizazi K, Shore N, Tammela TL, et al. Darolutamide in Nonmetastatic, Castration-Resistant Prostate Cancer. *New England Journal of Medicine* 2019;380(13):1235–46. PMID: 30763142.

Fizazi K, Shore N, Tammela TLA, et al. Nonmetastatic, Castration-Resistant Prostate Cancer and Survival with Darolutamide. *New England Journal of Medicine* 2020;383(11):1040–49. PMID: 32905676.

Hussain M, Fizazi K, Saad F, et al. Enzalutamide in Men with Nonmetastatic, Castration-Resistant Prostate Cancer. *New England Journal of Medicine* 2018;378(26):2465–74. PMID: 29949494.

Kumar J, Jazayeri SB, Gautam S, et al. Comparative Efficacy of Apalutamide, Darolutamide, and Enzalutamide for Treatment of Non-Metastatic Castrate-Resistant Prostate Cancer: A Systematic Review and Network Meta-Analysis. *Urologic Oncology* 2020;38(11):826–34. PMID: 32605736.

Loriot Y, Fizazi K, de Bono JS, et al. Enzalutamide in Castration-Resistant Prostate Cancer Patients with Visceral Disease in the Liver and/or Lung: Outcomes from the Randomized Controlled Phase 3 AFFIRM Trial. *Cancer* 2017;123(2):253–62. PMID: 27648814.

continued on page 82

factors such as high blood pressure. People with inflammatory bowel disease can also suffer a relapse. (For reference, see "Side effects of hormonal therapy," below left.)

Sexual dysfunction. Because hormonal therapy interferes with testosterone, sexual function is often a casualty of this type of treatment. Most men experience erectile dysfunction and a loss of sexual desire. When treatment is stopped, however, sexual function usually returns, especially in younger men who have received treatment for less than two years. Moreover, research indicates that men who exercise when starting hormonal therapy report fewer sexual side effects, more energy, and less tendency toward depression. (For reference, see "Hormonal therapy and sexual dysfunction," bottom left.)

Bone disease. Bone disease may develop in men with advanced prostate cancer for two reasons. First, one of the side effects of hormonal therapy is loss of bone tissue. Second, when prostate cancer spreads, it almost always spreads to the bone. Complications of prostate cancer in the bone (bone metastases) include pain, bone thinning, fractures, and spinal compression. Typically, these problems have been treated with pain medication and either radiation or surgery to stabilize the bone.

Until recently, just two drugs were available to help prevent fractures by building bone mass in men with prostate cancer—zoledronic acid (Zometa) and pamidronate disodium (Aredia). These drugs, called bisphosphonates, directly target osteoclasts, the cells that break down bone. The bisphosphonates are most commonly used to treat osteoporosis, the weakening of bone that often occurs in old age.

A newer drug, denosumab (Xgeva), works in a different way. It blocks a substance known as a RANK ligand, which is necessary to activate the bone-destroying osteoclasts. By blocking the RANK ligand, denosumab prevents bone erosion. The FDA approved denosumab in 2010 for men whose cancer had spread to the bone, after a study found that the drug increased bone density and reduced the risk of spinal fractures by more than half in prostate cancer patients. A year later, that approval was expanded to include treatment of men at risk for bone fractures because they are taking hormonal therapy for advanced prostate cancer.

A 2020 review paper concluded that denosumab was safe and effective for the prevention and management of bone side effects in men who were taking hormonal therapy for prostate cancer. Research published in 2021 showed that giving denosumab or zoledronic acid to build bone mass also improves survival in men with mCRPC who are being treated with abiraterone. (For references, see "Hormonal therapy and bone disease," page 83.)

Still, men taking any of these bone-preserving drugs are at risk for a rare dental complication, so you should see a dentist before taking any of them (see "Protecting your teeth and jawbone," page 83). Moreover, unusual fractures of the femur (thighbone) have been reported in patients taking bisphosphonates.

Cardiovascular risks. Hormonal therapy for prostate cancer can increase total cholesterol and triglyceride levels, as well as blood sugar levels. All these changes can potentially increase your risk of developing diabetes and cardiovascular disease, which is the leading cause of non-cancer death in men with prostate cancer. In 2021, the American Heart Association issued a statement recommending that men

Anti-androgens

continued from page 81

Saad F, Cella D, Basch E, et al. Effect of Apalutamide on Health-Related Quality of Life in Patients with Non-Metastatic Castration-Resistant Prostate Cancer: An Analysis of the SPARTAN Randomised, Placebo-Controlled, Phase 3 Trial. *Lancet Oncology* 2018;19(10):1404–16. PMID: 30213449.

Smith MR, Saad F, Chowdhury S, et al. Apalutamide Treatment and Metastasis-Free Survival in Prostate Cancer. *New England Journal of Medicine* 2018;378(15):1408–18. PMID: 29420164.

Abiraterone and enzalutamide

Davis ID, Martin AJ, Stockler MR, et al. Enzalutamide with Standard First-Line Therapy in Metastatic Prostate Cancer. *New England Journal of Medicine* 2019;381(2):121–31. PMID: 31157964.

Fizazi K, Tran N, Fein L, et al. Abiraterone plus Prednisone in Metastatic, Castration-Sensitive Prostate Cancer. *New England Journal of Medicine* 2017;377(4):352–60. PMID: 28578607.

Matsubara N, Yamada Y, Tabata KI, et al. Abiraterone Followed by Enzalutamide Versus Enzalutamide Followed by Abiraterone in Chemotherapy-Naive Patients with Metastatic Castration-Resistant Prostate Cancer. *Clinical Genitourinary Cancer* 2018;16(2):142–48. PMID: 29042308.

Mori K, Miura N, Mostafaei H, et al. Sequential Therapy of Abiraterone and Enzalutamide in Castration-Resistant Prostate Cancer: A Systematic Review and Meta-Analysis. *Prostate Cancer and Prostatic Diseases* 2020; 23(4):539–48. PMID: 32152435.

Side effects of hormonal therapy

Axelrod JE, Bazarbashi A, Zhou J, et al. Hormone Therapy for Cancer is a Risk Factor for Relapse of Inflammatory Bowel Disease. *Clinical Gasteroenterology and Hepatology* 2020;18(4):872–80. PMID: 31302306.

Hormonal therapy and sexual dysfunction

Cormie P, Galvão DA, Spry N, et al. Can Supervised Exercise Prevent Treatment Toxicity in Patients with Prostate Cancer Initiating Androgen-Deprivation Therapy: A Randomised Controlled Trial. *BJU International* 2015;115(2):256–66. PMID: 24467669.

undergoing hormonal therapy for prostate cancer should be closely monitored for potential cardiovascular complications, especially if they already have risk factors such as high blood pressure, high cholesterol, smoking, and a family history of heart disease. These complications are increasingly grouped together in a category known as major adverse cardiovascular events (MACE), including heart attacks, strokes, or death from a heart-related cause. Before starting hormonal therapy, ask your doctor to measure your blood sugar, blood pressure, and cholesterol levels and to perform an electrocardiogram. (For references, see "Hormonal therapy and cardiovascular disease," page 84.)

Liver disease. A study published in 2018 provided new evidence linking hormonal therapy with liver disease. The investigators reviewed national cancer registry data for a total of 82,938 men who were diagnosed with localized prostate cancer between 1992 and 2009. Of them, just over 31,000 were treated with ADT, and those men were 54% more likely than the men who were not given hormonal therapy to be diagnosed subsequently with nonalcoholic liver disease. Moreover, ADT significantly increased risks for liver cirrhosis, liver necrosis, and other types of liver disease. The likelihood of developing these conditions rose as the duration of hormonal therapy increased. (For reference, see "Hormonal therapy and liver disease," page 84.)

Anti-androgens such as bicalutamide, in rare cases, cause a condition called transaminitis, characterized by high blood levels of certain liver enzymes known as transaminases. Dr. Garnick checks liver function every two weeks during the first eight weeks of anti-androgen therapy, since this is when liver injury from treatment is most likely to occur. If left untreated, transaminitis can result in severe liver injury and possibly death.

Cognitive decline. Low testosterone levels have been associated with a higher risk for dementia, and a study in 2019 suggested that hormonal therapy may pose a similar risk. The researchers looked at data on 154,089 men with prostate cancer, including 62,330 who were treated with hormonal therapy and 91,759 who were not. The results showed a slightly higher risk of dementia after 10 years. But the authors cautioned that they were unable to consider other strong predictors for cognitive decline, such as family history, high blood pressure, or head injuries. And a 2021 study found no evidence of cognitive decline in men with mCRPC who were being treated with either enzalutamide or abiraterone (see "Study finds no cognitive impact from treatment for advanced prostate cancer," page 9; for references, see "Hormonal therapy and cognitive decline," page 85.)

Combined hormonal therapy and radiation therapy

Hormonal therapy is sometimes given in conjunction with external beam radiation to boost the effectiveness of treatment. Hormonal therapy may also be used to shrink large prostate glands (typically defined as those weighing more than 50 grams) before brachytherapy takes place, to enable proper placement of the radioactive seeds.

Combination hormonal/radiation therapy is now a standard option for men with cancer that has extended beyond the prostate (stage T3 or T4) or whose cancer is considered high-risk based on other clinical findings, with studies showing that

Hormonal therapy and bone disease

Francini E, Montagnani F, Nuzzo PV, et al. Association of Concomitant Bone Resorption Inhibitors with Overall Survival Among Patients with Metastatic Castration-Resistant Prostate Cancer and Bone Metastases Receiving Abiraterone Acetate with Prednisone as First-Line Therapy. *JAMA Network Open* 2021;4(7):e2116536. PMID: 34292336.

Walz S, Maas M, Stenzl A, et al. Bone Health Issues in Patients with Prostate Cancer: An Evidence-Based Review. *World Journal of Men's Health* 2020:38(2):151–63. PMID: 31081297.

PubMed See page 120.

Protecting your teeth and jawbone

The bone agents used to help men with prostate cancer can cause a rare but distressing problem known as osteonecrosis of the jaw, in which the jawbone dies after its blood supply is cut off. It is not clear who might develop this condition, although men who undergo invasive dental work—such as tooth extraction—while taking a bone-preserving agent seem to be more at risk. For that reason, it is important to see your dentist for a check-up, and consider having any tooth or jaw problems treated, before starting a bone drug. While taking bone drugs, exercise good dental hygiene, continue seeing your dentist for check-ups, and report to your physicians any episodes of pain in the mouth and jaw area.

it reduces the risk of dying from prostate cancer and other causes more than either treatment given alone.

Studies have shown that long-term hormonal treatment is better than short-term treatments lasting a few months for patients in the high-risk category who are also treated with high-dose radiation. Along those lines, scientists reported results from a study in 2017 showing that patients who have locally advanced prostate cancer should receive hormonal therapy for at least two years after radiotherapy. The study launched in 1992 and enrolled approximately 1,500 men with cancer that had spread into nearby tissues, such as the bladder. The data show that after 20 years, men who got the long-term treatment had a 29% lower risk of dying from prostate cancer as well as a 46% lower risk of metastasis than those who were given hormonal therapy for just four months. Based on these results, Dr. Garnick says two years of hormonal therapy should now be strongly considered.

Research also shows that hormonal therapy and radiation given together is more effective than radiation by itself at treating prostate cancer that returns after radical prostatectomy. A study published in 2019 demonstrated that 10-year survival was significantly better among men who had a combination of salvage radiation (radiation given when cancer returns after radical prostatectomy) and the LHRH agonist goserelin compared with those who got radiation alone.

A study published in 2021 supports the use of combination therapy for patients at the higher end of the intermediate-risk category. The results showed that six months of hormonal therapy slowed cancer progression among men with intermediate-risk disease, although the effects on overall survival were inconclusive. (For a quick assessment of risk profiles, see Table 4, page 59.) Whether men with low-risk prostate cancer would benefit from a combination of hormonal therapy and radiation is uncertain. Combined treatment is more likely than radiation alone to cause erectile dysfunction—and some research suggests that the problem may be less responsive to intervention to improve erectile function after treatment. The research is conflicting about whether any of these side effects persists in the long term. Until more is known, be aware that side effects do occur with combined therapy and that it's important to discuss this issue with your doctor. (For references, see "Combined hormonal therapy and radiation therapy," page 85.)

Combined hormonal therapy and chemotherapy

In 2015, results from a trial sponsored by the National Cancer Institute (NCI) showed that men with metastatic prostate cancer lived longer if they started chemotherapy along with hormonal therapy instead of going on hormonal therapy by itself. Men with the most advanced cancers benefited most from the combination: they lived roughly 49 months, or 17 months longer than men who were started on ADT alone. The trial investigators, noting the side effects of chemotherapy, cautioned that the hormonal therapy–chemotherapy combination should be used only in patients with high-volume cancer (occupying more than 25% of the prostate gland) that is also metastatic.

Hormonal therapy and cardiovascular disease

Butler SS, Mahal BA, Moslehi, et al. Risk of Cardiovascular Mortality with Androgen Deprivation Therapy in Prostate Cancer: A Secondary Analysis of the Prostate, Lung, Colorectal, and Ovarian (PLCO) Randomized Controlled Trial. *Cancer* 2021;127(13):2213–21. PMID: 33905530.

Gupta D, Lee Chuy K, Yang JC, et al. Cardiovascular and Metabolic Effects of Androgen-Deprivation Therapy for Prostate Cancer. *Journal of Oncology Practice* 2018;14(10):580–87. PMID: 30312560.

Kelly WK, Gomella LG. Androgen Deprivation Therapy and Competing Risks. *JAMA* 2011;306(21):2382–83. PMID: 22147384.

Nguyen PL, Je Y, Schutz FA, et al. Association of Androgen Deprivation Therapy with Cardiovascular Death in Patients with Prostate Cancer: A Meta-Analysis of Randomized Trials. *JAMA* 2011;306(21):2359–66. PMID: 22147380.

Okwuosa TM, Morgans A, Rhee JW, et al. Impact of Hormonal Therapies for Treatment of Hormone-Dependent Cancers (Breast and Prostate) on the Cardiovascular System: Effects and Modifications: A Scientific Statement from the American Heart Association. *Circulation: Genomic and Precision Medicine* 2021;14(3):e000082. PMID: 33896190.

Salem JE, Yang T, Moslehi JJ, et al. Androgenic Effects on Ventricular Repolarization: A Translational Study from the International Pharmacovigilance Database to iPSC-Cardiomyocytes. *Circulation* 2019;140(13):1070–80. PMID: 31378084.

Tivesten Å, Pinthus JH, Clarke N, et al. Cardiovascular Risk with Androgen Deprivation Therapy for Prostate Cancer: Potential Mechanisms. *Urologic Oncology* 2015;33(11):464–75. PMID: 26141678.

Hormonal therapy and liver disease

Gild P, Cole AP, Krasnova A, et al. Liver Disease in Men Undergoing Androgen Deprivation Therapy for Prostate Cancer. *Journal of Urology* 2018;200(3):573–81. PMID: 29673944.

Other researchers have also found survival advantages from the combined therapy. The ongoing STAMPEDE study, for instance, is similarly evaluating outcomes in men diagnosed with either metastatic or high-risk prostate cancer who receive ADT by itself or following upfront use of docetaxel, the main drug used in chemotherapy for prostate cancer. An analysis published in 2016, when 3,000 men were participating in the study, showed that men given ADT alone survived 71 months, while those who took docetaxel and hormonal therapy lived 81 months. An updated analysis of the STAMPEDE study published in 2019 showed that men given the combined treatment still had a survival advantage over men who were treated with hormonal therapy by itself.

As for quality of life, men receiving the combined treatment in the NCI study had more side effects than those receiving hormonal therapy alone, and that raised concerns. But results from the STAMPEDE study revealed those side effects were transient—within six months, most patients receiving the combined treatment felt almost back to normal, and within a year, they felt as they had before the treatment. In fact, some of the men treated with combined therapy reported better quality-of-life measures over time than those treated with hormonal therapy alone.

That said, some men have difficulty tolerating docetaxel, so doctors might also consider a multitude of other, potentially less toxic therapies that were not available when the NCI study was launched. Most clinicians agree that the combined treatment is more appropriate for men who can tolerate chemotherapy, meaning individuals who are not old, frail, or sick with other potentially life-threatening conditions.

Researchers had speculated that combining docetaxel with hormonal therapy might be similarly beneficial for men with rising PSA levels after initial treatment

Intermittent vs. continuous hormonal therapy

Hormonal therapy can be delivered either continuously or with periodic breaks in treatment, an approach known as intermittent hormonal therapy. The regimens vary, but the basic plan is to stop hormonal therapy once a man's PSA falls below a certain level and then start up therapy again if his PSA starts to increase. The rationale is that on-again, off-again treatment may make hormonal therapy more effective by making prostate cancer cells more sensitive to the withdrawal of testosterone and related hormones. Intermittent therapy also gives men a "drug holiday" from the side effects of hormonal therapy.

A number of large studies have compared intermittent with continuous hormonal therapy, but the jury is still out. A review published in 2019 concluded that there is not enough evidence to assess what impact intermittent therapy might have on metastatic disease progression and survival and that the data so far suggest only modest benefits for quality of life and symptom relief in the short term. Dr. Garnick urges extreme caution in using intermittent hormonal therapy in patients with metastatic disease, since some studies have shown better results with continuous hormonal therapy.

Sources: Hussain M, Tangen CM, Berry DL, et al. Intermittent Versus Continuous Androgen Deprivation in Prostate Cancer. *New England Journal of Medicine* 2013;368(14):1314–25. PMID: 23550669.

Shevach J, Sydes MR, Hussain M. Revisiting Intermittent Therapy in Metastatic Prostate Cancer: Can Less be More in the "New World Order"? *European Urology Focus* 2019;5(2):125–33. PMID: 30803926.

Hormonal therapy and cognitive decline

Alibhai SMH, Breunis H, Feng G, et al. Association of Chemotherapy, Enzalutamide, Abiraterone, and Radium 223 with Cognitive Function in Older Men with Metastatic Castration-Resistant Prostate Cancer. *JAMA Network Open* 2021;4(7):e2114694. PMID: 34213559.

Jayadevappa R, Chhatre S, Malkowicz SB, et al. Association Between Androgen Deprivation Therapy Use and Diagnosis of Dementia in Men with Prostate Cancer. *JAMA Network Open* 2019;2(27):e196562. PMID: 31268539.

Combined hormonal therapy and radiation therapy

Boevé L, Hulshof MCCM, Verhagen PCMS, et al. Patient-Reported Quality of Life in Patients with Primary Metastatic Prostate Cancer Treated with Androgen Deprivation Therapy With and Without Concurrent Radiation Therapy to the Prostate in a Prospective Randomised Clinical Trial: Data from the HORRAD Trial. *European Urology* 2021;79(2):188–97. PMID: 32978014.

Bolla M, Neven A, Maingon P, et al. Short Androgen Suppression and Radiation Dose Escalation in Prostate Cancer: 12-Year Results of the EORTC Trial 22991 in Patients with Localized Intermediate-Risk Disease. *Journal of Clinical Oncology* 2021;39(27):3022–33. PMID: 34310202.

Carrie C, Magné N, Burban-Provost P, et al. Interest of Short Hormonotherapy (HT) Associated with Radiotherapy (RT) as Salvage Treatment for Metastatic Free Survival (MFS) after Radical Prostatectomy (RP): Update at 9 Years of the GETUG-AFU 16 Phase III Randomized Trial (NCT00423475). *Journal of Clinical Oncology* 2019;20(12):1740–49. PMID: 31629656.

Lawton CAF, Lin X, Hanks GE, et al. Duration of Androgen Deprivation in Locally Advanced Prostate Cancer: Long-Term Update of NRG Oncology RTOG 9202. *International Journal of Radiation Oncology, Biology, Physics* 2017;98(2):296–303. PMID: 28463149.

PubMed See page 120.

with surgery or radiation. But results from a study with 250 men that was published in 2019 were disappointing. After just over 10 years of follow-up, there were no differences in subsequent PSA levels or quality of life among men who were treated with docetaxel and hormonal therapy or with hormonal therapy alone. The authors claimed that comparing PSA changes was appropriate since levels rise in tandem with disease progression. (For references, see "Combined hormonal therapy and chemotherapy," at left.)

Chemotherapy

Although it's often a standard treatment for other cancers, chemotherapy up until recently was rarely used to treat early prostate cancer because prostate tumors typically grow slowly. (Chemotherapy targets cells that proliferate rapidly.) It is used, though, to treat advanced cases of the disease that are no longer responding to other treatments. Chemotherapy drugs for prostate cancer are given intravenously. They are usually taken in cycles, with each period of treatment followed by an off period.

Docetaxel is the mainstay of the chemotherapy drugs used to treat advanced prostate cancer (see Table 8, page 87). The FDA approved another drug, cabazitaxel (Jevtana), in 2011. Like docetaxel, cabazitaxel is in the taxane class of chemotherapy drugs. Cabazitaxel is effective in many men whose cancers have become resistant to other drugs in the taxane family. However, it is associated with significant side effects, including reduced numbers of blood cells in bone marrow.

Side effects

Because chemotherapy drugs are absorbed by tissues throughout the body, healthy cells can also be harmed, especially those that are dividing quickly. Hair loss, one of the classic side effects of chemotherapy, occurs because the drugs damage the dividing cells of hair follicles. Cells in the bone marrow, mouth, stomach, tear ducts, and intestines are also commonly affected. Both toenails and fingernails can also be affected and sometimes fall off.

Aside from hair loss, chemotherapy may cause fatigue, mouth sores, nausea, gastrointestinal disturbances, and infertility. The presence or absence of side effects, however, doesn't show how well the therapy is working. Most men find the side effects manageable, and the effects don't last very long. In a few months, the chemotherapy is finished, their bodies recover, and they steadily return to feeling normal.

PARP inhibitors

All cells experience routine genetic damage. They have various mechanisms to repair it, including a set of enzymes called poly (ADP-ribose) polymerases, or PARPs. When cancer cells repair the damage, they can continue growing and replicating. Drugs known as PARP inhibitors prevent cancer cells from making these repairs. The damage therefore accumulates until the cells die. PARP inhibitors were developed initially for treating BRCA-positive breast and ovarian cancers in women. But BRCA muta-

continued on page 88

Combined hormonal therapy and chemotherapy

Clarke NW, Ali A, Ingleby FC, et al. Addition of Docetaxel to Hormonal Therapy in Low- and High-Burden Metastatic Hormone Sensitive Prostate Cancer: Long-Term Survival Results from the STAMPEDE Trial. *Annals of Oncology* 2019;30(12):1992–2003. PMID: 31560068.

Gravis G, Fizazi K, Joly F, et al. Androgen-Deprivation Therapy Alone or with Docetaxel in Non-Castrate Metastatic Prostate Cancer (GETUG-AFU 15): A Randomised, Open-Label, Phase 3 Trial. *Lancet Oncology* 2013;14(2):149–58. PMID: 23306100.

James ND, Sydes MR, Clarke NW, et al. Addition of Docetaxel, Zoledronic Acid, or Both to First-Line Long-Term Hormone Therapy in Prostate Cancer (STAMPEDE): Survival Results from an Adaptive, Multiarm, Multistage, Platform Randomised Controlled Trial. *Lancet* 2016;387(10024):1163–77. PMID: 26719232.

Oudard S, Latorzeff I, Caty A, et al. Effect of Adding Docetaxel to Androgen-Deprivation Therapy in Patients with High-Risk Prostate Cancer with Rising Prostate-Specific Antigen Levels After Primary Local Therapy: A Randomized Clinical Trial. *JAMA Oncology* 2019;5(5):623–32. PMID: 30703190.

Sweeney CJ, Chen YH, Carducci M, et al. Chemohormonal Therapy in Metastatic Hormone-Sensitive Prostate Cancer. *New England Journal of Medicine* 2015;373(8):737–46. PMID 26244877.

Woods BS, Sideris E, Sydes MR, et al. Addition of Docetaxel to First-line Long-term Hormone Therapy in Prostate Cancer (STAMPEDE): Modelling to Estimate Long-term Survival, Quality-adjusted Survival, and Cost-effectiveness. *European Urology Oncology* 2018;1(6):449–58. PMID: 31158087.

PubMed See page 120.

Table 8. Chemotherapy, targeted therapy (PARP inhibitors), and immunotherapy for advanced prostate cancer

Drug name	Common side effects	Comments
Standard chemotherapy (FDA-approved for prostate cancer)		
cabazitaxel (Jevtana)	Drop in blood cell counts, diarrhea, fatigue, nausea, vomiting, constipation, weakness, kidney failure.	In combination with the steroid prednisone, cabazitaxel is approved for use in men who no longer respond to docetaxel. It can extend survival.
docetaxel (Taxotere)	Hair loss, nausea and vomiting, drop in blood cell counts, numbness and tingling (usually in the feet).	This anti-cancer drug may be used alone or in combination with other chemotherapeutic agents, such as estramustine and carboplatin. It may also be used initially with hormonal therapy for men with extensive metastases. Docetaxel can extend survival.
Chemotherapy used "off label" (not specifically approved for prostate cancer)		
carboplatin (Paraplatin)	Low blood cell counts, nausea, vomiting, taste changes, hair loss, weakness, constipation, diarrhea.	Used as a single agent and in combination with paclitaxel and estramustine. Also used as a second-line therapy for patients who have become resistant to docetaxel. Although not specifically approved for the treatment of prostate cancer, it can ease symptoms.
paclitaxel (Taxol)	Hair loss, nausea and vomiting, fatigue, drop in blood cell counts, numbness and tingling in hands and feet (usually after long-term use).	Although not specifically approved for the treatment of prostate cancer, it can ease symptoms.
Other chemotherapy drugs		
estramustine (Emcyt)	Blood clots, nausea and vomiting, fatigue, headache, drop in blood cell counts.	Often combined with other agents in clinical trials, but the risk of blood clots and other complications make estramustine unlikely to become a standard treatment. Approved for use in prostate cancer patients to ease symptoms.
mitoxantrone (Novantrone)	Nausea and vomiting, hair loss, fatigue, drop in blood cell counts.	This drug is often used in men who do not respond to docetaxel; eases symptoms.
PARP inhibitors (FDA-approved for prostate cancer)		
olaparib (Lynparza)	Decreased hemoglobin, nausea, fatigue, drop in white blood cell count, abdominal pain, vomiting, anemia.	Used in men with a BRCA gene mutation to reduce PSA levels, shrink tumors, lessen pain, and improve quality of life.
rucaparib (Rubraca)	Fatigue, vomiting, nausea, anemia, drop in white blood cell count.	Used to extend survival in men with a BRCA gene mutation who no longer respond to other treatments.
Immunotherapy		
pembrolizumab (Keytruda)	Fatigue, cough, nausea, itching, rash, shortness of breath, pericarditis, colitis.	May help men whose tumors contain mutated mismatch repair genes.
sipuleucel-T (Provenge)	Fever, chills, fatigue, back pain, nausea, joint pain, headache.	Extends survival for men with minimally metastatic disease. Data have been controversial and drug does not induce a measurable clinical response.

Note: This is a partial list, reflecting the more promising chemotherapeutic agents in clinical practice and in clinical trials. It does not include all agents or those in early stages of development. Those that have not been approved by the FDA for the treatment of prostate cancer might not be covered by health insurance.

PARP inhibitors

Abida W, Patnaik A, Campbell D, et al. Rucaparib in Men with Metastatic Castration-Resistant Prostate Cancer Harboring a BRCA1 or BRCA2 Gene Alteration. *Journal of Clinical Oncology* 2020;38(32):3763–72. PMID: 32795228.

De Bono J, Mateo J, Fizazi K, et al. Olaparib for Metastatic Castration-Resistant Prostate Cancer. *New England Journal of Medicine* 2020;382(22):2091–102. PMID: 32343890.

Radium-223

Parker CC, Coleman RE, Sartor O, et al. Three-Year Safety of Radium-223 Dichloride in Patients with Castration-Resistant Prostate Cancer and Symptomatic Bone Metastases from Phase 3 Randomized Alpharadin in Symptomatic Prostate Cancer Trial. *European Urology* 2018;73(3):427–35. PMID: 28705540.

Parker C, Nilsson S, Heinrich D, et al. Alpha Emitter Radium-223 and Survival in Metastatic Prostate Cancer. *New England Journal of Medicine* 2013;369(3):213–23. PMID: 23863050.

Saad F, Carles J, Gillessen S. Radium-223 and Concomitant Therapies in Patients with Metastatic Castration-Resistant Prostate Cancer: An International, Early Access, Open-Label, Single Arm Phase 3B Trial. *Lancet Oncology* 2016;17(9):1306–16. PMID: 27473888.

Smith M, Parker C, Saad F, et al. Addition of Radium 223 to Abiraterone Acetate and Prednisone or Prednisolone in Patients with Castration-Resistant Prostate Cancer and Bone Metastases (ERA 223): A Randomised, Double-Blind, Placebo-Controlled, Phase 3 Trial. *Lancet Oncology* 2019;20(3):408–19. PMID: 30738780.

Tosco L, Devos G, Schillebeeckx L, et al. Radium-223 in Patients with Prostate Specific Antigen (PSA) Progression and Without Clinical Metastases Following Maximal Local Therapy: A Pilot Study. *Urologic Oncology* 2022;40(1):7.c9–17. PMID: 34099385.

continued from page 86

tions are also strong risk factors for aggressive prostate cancer in men. About 10% of men with metastatic prostate cancer test positive for these mutations.

In 2020, the FDA approved a pair of PARP inhibitors specifically for BRCA-positive prostate tumors that no longer respond to other treatments—olaparib (Lynparza) and rucaparib (Rubraca). The approvals mark a major advance for targeted prostate cancer therapies given to genetically defined populations with few other treatment options. During the clinical trial leading to rucaparib's approval, tumors shrank in 44% of treated men for up to two years. Olaparib similarly delayed cancer progression for an average of 7.4 months, which was just over twice as long as the delay achieved with ADT in the control group. (For references, see "PARP inhibitors," at left.)

Bone-targeting treatments

When prostate cancer metastasizes, it spreads to the bone about 90% of the time. Often prostate cancer's most serious—and sometimes deadliest—consequences are those involving bone tissue, including a higher risk of fractures and associated complications. Thus, one promising strategy for treating prostate cancer is to control the disease once it has entered bone tissue.

The FDA approved radium-223 (Xofigo) in May 2013. Xofigo attacks prostate cancer lurking in bone by exposing it to high-energy alpha-particle radiation that is attracted to areas of the bone affected by cancer. Results of an industry-sponsored trial were published in 2013. The main outcome was that men with metastatic cancer who received radium-223 lived longer than men who received the placebo (14.9 months vs. 11.3 months). That may seem like a small difference, but these men had advanced prostate disease with a high fatality rate, so even small survival gains are important.

The FDA approved radium-223 for the treatment of men with advanced prostate cancer that has spread to the bone, not to other organs, and only after efforts to control the prostate cancer with hormones have failed. For a new study published in 2021, researchers investigated using the drug to limit bone metastases in men with rising PSA levels after initial treatment. Results showed the treatment was safe and well tolerated, but clinical benefits from this strategy are uncertain. Another study, which examined the use of radium-223 plus abiraterone versus abiraterone plus a placebo had the unexpected finding that the combination incurred a higher rate of fractures and a lower overall survival rate. These findings have now been incorporated into warnings recommending against the concurrent use of these two agents. (For references, see "Radium-223," at left.)

Immunotherapy

Immunotherapies (or cancer "vaccines") turn the body's own immune system against tumor cells and have proven successful in many different types of cancer. But in prostate cancer, the drugs have met with limited success. An FDA-approved cancer vaccine for prostate cancer, sipuleucel-T (Provenge), doesn't induce a measurable clinical response, such as a decline in PSA, making its effects difficult for doctors to monitor.

That said, a 2020 review of Medicare claims data from 6,044 men treated for mCRPC detected a survival advantage from sipuleucel-T. Results showed that men who received the immunotherapy lived 14 months longer on average than those who did not. However, insurance claims data contain limited clinical information and are therefore less informative than clinical trials.

Other immunotherapy drugs are showing promise. One called pembrolizumab (Keytruda) was approved by the FDA in 2017 for all metastatic cancers that test positive for mutations affecting the mismatch repair (MMR) genes, which ordinarily patch the DNA damage that occurs routinely when cells divide. As DNA damage accumulates, cells can become genetically unstable, and cancer often results. To protect themselves, cancer cells rely on proteins called checkpoints that can deflect an incoming attack by the immune system. Pembrolizumab is a checkpoint inhibitor that disables this protective mechanism.

A study published in 2019 tested pembrolizumab in prostate cancer patients whose tumors contained MMR defects. In nearly half of the treated men, PSA levels dropped over 50%. And in approximately 40% of the PSA responders, tumors also shrank visibly. Dr. Garnick recommends that all patients with metastatic cancer be tested for MMR defects since they may respond to pembrolizumab or other checkpoint-inhibiting drugs.

Another drug, called ipilimumab (Yervoy), which is approved by the FDA for melanoma and other cancers, inactivates a protein called CTLA-4 that protects tumors from the immune system. (For references, see "Immunotherapy," at right.)

Immunotherapy

Abida W, Cheng ML, Armenia J, et al. Analysis of the Prevalence of Microsatellite Instability in Prostate Cancer and Response to Immune Checkpoint Blockade. *JAMA Oncology* 2019;5(4):471–78. PMID: 30589920.

Higano CS, Armstrong AJ, Sartor AO, et al. Real-World Outcomes of Sipuleucel-T Treatment in PROCEED, a Prospective Registry of Men with Metastatic Castration-Resistant Prostate Cancer. *Cancer* 2019;125(23):4172–80. PMID: 31483485.

McKay RR, Hafron JM, Ferro C, et al. A Retrospective Observational Analysis of Overall Survival with Sipuleucel-T in Medicare Beneficiaries Treated for Advanced Prostate Cancer. *Advanced Therapeutics* 2020;37(12):4910–29. PMID: 33029725.

Reimers MA, Slane KE, Pachynski RK. Immunotherapy in Metastatic Castration-Resistant Prostate Cancer: Past and Future Strategies for Optimization. *Current Urology Reports* 2019;20(10):64. PMID: 31482315.

PubMed See page 120.

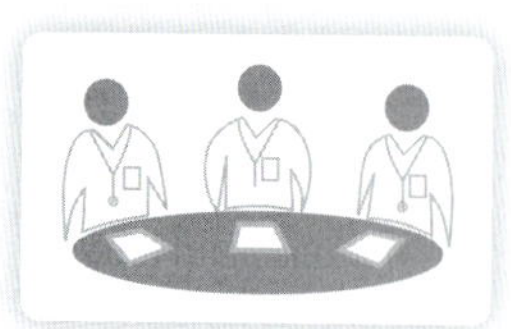

ROUNDTABLE DISCUSSION:

New hope in treating oligometastatic prostate cancer

Oligometastatic cancer is an early form of stage 4 prostate cancer that has spread to other organs in the body, but only to a limited degree—generally defined as no more than three to five areas outside the prostate gland, most commonly in the lymph nodes or bones. Barely a decade ago, it was considered universally fatal, and treatment was limited to hormonal therapy. But now, exciting developments in the field are leading to new treatment strategies that are improving patient survival in clinical trials. Together with better, earlier detection of oligometastatic cancer—made possible with new imaging agents such as fluciclovine (Axumin) and gallium-68—this could even lead to cures in small subsets of patients, a concept that was unimaginable as recently as 10 years ago.

To help our readers better understand the complex issues in this rapidly developing field, we convened an expert panel for a wide-ranging discussion of the biology and evolving methods for treating the disease. Our panel includes specialists in prostate cancer surgery, medical oncology, and radiation oncology.

Nima Aghdam, M.D., is a radiation oncologist at Beth Israel Deaconess Medical Center (BIDMC) in Boston. He specializes in genitourinary malignancies with a special focus on the role of stereotactic body radiation therapy in the management of localized and oligometastatic prostate cancer.

Anthony D'Amico, M.D., is a professor of radiation oncology at Harvard Medical School and chief of genitourinary radiation oncology at Brigham and Women's Hospital and Dana-Farber Cancer Institute. He has gained international recognition for his work in detection, staging, and treatment of prostate cancer, with over 140 peer-reviewed publications, and has co-edited four textbooks on urologic oncology.

David J. Einstein, M.D., is a medical oncologist specializing in genitourinary cancers, an attending physician at BIDMC, and assistant professor of medicine at Harvard Medical School. He focuses on the testing of new treatments and is the overall principal investigator for prostate cancer trials taking place through the Dana-Farber/Harvard Cancer Center research consortium.

Boris Gershman, M.D., is a urologic surgeon at BIDMC and assistant professor of surgery at Harvard Medical School. His clinical interests focus on the management of prostate, kidney, bladder, and testicular cancer. His research interests include a subspecialty of urologic oncology known as comparative effectiveness and health services research. He also serves as a reviewer for multiple medical journals.

Cora N. Sternberg, M.D., F.A.C.P., is a medical oncologist and professor of medicine at Weill Cornell Medicine and NewYork-Presbyterian Hospital. Her research specialties are bladder cancer, prostate cancer, and renal cell carcinoma. She has published six textbooks and more than 400 research articles and is an editorial board member of several international journals.

Marc B. Garnick, M.D., editor in chief of the *Annual,* moderated the discussion.

Q: What's the definition of oligometastatic disease?
D'Amico: Simply put, it's prostate cancer with a limited number of sites of metastases—some experts say three, others five. Those sites can be in bone, where prostate cancer often travels, or in the lymph nodes, or in organs like the liver or lungs. The condition has also been defined as at most three sites of metastasis, but where all the positive lymph nodes count as a single site. So, one positive node or a bunch of them—either way, according to this alternate definition, that's one site. And the lymph node disease can be extensive in the body, or very limited.

Q: Which definition do you think is most appropriate?
D'Amico: Well, I think three sites of metastases is reasonable. But I would count multiple positive lymph nodes as a single site only if they were all in the same region—say, the pelvis, or abdomen, or chest.

Q: Why is it considered distinct from other stage 4 cancers?

ROUNDTABLE DISCUSSION *continued*

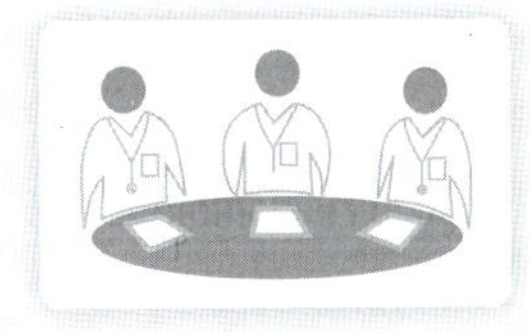

D'Amico: It has fewer metastases than other stage 4 cancers. Thanks to advances in screening, doctors are now able to find smaller deposits of malignant cells outside the prostate gland that were previously undetectable.

Q: What's the difference between de novo and oligorecurring prostate cancer?
Sternberg: De novo refers to newly diagnosed oligometastatic prostate cancer that hasn't been treated yet. Oligorecurring means the patient was treated for localized cancer in the prostate, and then went on to develop the metastases later.

Q: What about oligoprogressive disease?
Einstein: In this case, the primary tumor and the metastases are growing—but not becoming more widely disseminated—while a man is also being treated with systemic therapy. By that I mean drugs that target cancer throughout the body.
Sternberg: Keep in mind that oligoprogression sometimes occurs without changes to a man's PSA levels. So even though a man's PSA seems to be okay, he can still develop oligometastatic disease. For these men, new methods for diagnostic imaging are important for identifying the potential presence of cancer deposits in areas outside the prostate gland.

Q: Let's turn to the imaging advances that made oligometastatic disease a new entity. What do we use to diagnose it?
Einstein: We typically start with standard CT and MRI scans for cross-sectional views of the body. When scanning the bones, we inject a tracer that attaches to metastatic tumors, which we're then able to see with a device called a gamma camera. These standard approaches are widely used for initial staging, meaning the process by which we determine how much cancer is in the body when it's first diagnosed. But they aren't all that good at picking up early recurring cancer, because the tumors at that point are still too small to see with standard diagnostic imaging methods.

If we want to treat these small metastatic deposits, then we need to image them with better resolution. That's where positron emission tomography [PET] comes into the picture. PET scans also rely on tracers that have been developed specifically for prostate cancer. The one that's used most widely is an FDA-approved agent called fluciclovine, known commercially as Axumin. A newer tracer called gallium-68 is also generating a lot of excitement. It binds to a protein on cancer cells called prostate-specific membrane antigen [PSMA]. PSMA scanning is one of the more sensitive techniques for detecting small cancerous deposits outside the prostate gland. In the United States, it's approved for use at just two academic centers, both in California. And in May, the FDA approved a third tracer, piflufolastat F18, known commercially as Pylarify.
Gershman: Choline PET also has fairly limited availability in the United States.
Sternberg: I've had access to choline PET and found it was actually quite useful in picking up oligometastatic disease. We are testing PSMA scanning in clinical trials at Weill Cornell Medical right now.

Q: Could Axumin scans today serve as a substitute for standard imaging when you're working up a newly diagnosed patient for suspected metastases?
Sternberg: I don't think so. We use it under special circumstances when we're not really sure what we're seeing on MRI or CT, but generally not for initial scanning.
Aghdam: Same here. I use Axumin after PSA reaches a certain level, to look for recurrence.
Gershman: I would agree that for the initial workup in a newly diagnosed patient, it's not standard of care.
D'Amico: I concur, and that's because there isn't enough clinical trial evidence using biopsies to confirm suspected metastases picked up with Axumin PET. It's important to point out that even if an Axumin scan shows signs of metastasis, there's going to be some uncertainty about that unless you have a biopsy. I would lean toward using PSMA PET for initial staging only if we think a patient has a high or very high risk of metastatic cancer. But we still need more biopsy-proven data with PSMA, and a better understanding of how often the test generates false-positive results. Those studies are ongoing now.

Q: So why not do standard bone scans, abdominal/pelvic CT,* and *Axumin scanning until PSMA becomes

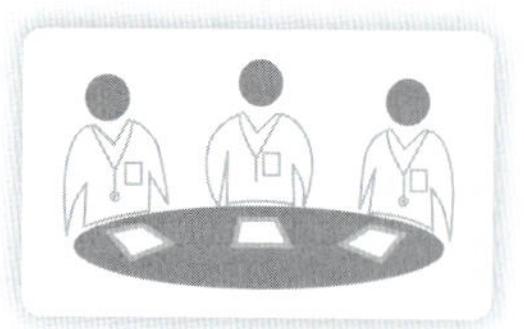

ROUNDTABLE DISCUSSION *continued*

more widely available? Couldn't we do all three of these studies for initial staging at once?

D'Amico: I'll give you two answers. One is that insurance will probably not pay for it. And again, from a medical standpoint, we still need more biopsy proof that what we see on an Axumin PET is more definitively positive than what we see on standard imaging. We don't want to exclude someone from potentially curative therapy [below] based on ambiguous PET findings.

Q: Moving on to therapy now, how do we treat the metastases?

Einstein: Usually we do it with stereotactic body radiation therapy [SBRT], but other approaches may be possible too. We can remove positive lymph nodes surgically, for instance. We can use radiofrequency ablation, which uses heat made by radio waves to kill cells, or cryoablation, which is a method for destroying cancerous tissue by freezing it.

Q: What can you tell us about SBRT?

Aghdam: This is a catch-all term that includes a number of precision techniques for delivering high-dose radiation to very small targets with imaging to guide you. We call a day's dose of radiation a "fraction," and with SBRT we're aiming to give only a few fractions, but with doses high enough to control the disease, and possibly cure it. Here in the United States, we generally give SBRT over the course of five fractions at most.

D'Amico: That way, a course of radiation treatment that would ordinarily take six to nine weeks can be done in two weeks or less.

Q: And the side effects?

Aghdam: SBRT has a relatively good side effects profile. But radiation in any dose causes fatigue for patients. Since we're trying to eradicate the cancer completely, we anticipate a certain degree of risk to normal tissues surrounding the radiation target. Patients can experience more frequent urination and bowel movements following radiation to the prostate, for instance. Targeting bone metastases can increase the risk of skeletal fracture, especially with the highest-dose treatments. In general, treating oligometastatic tumors presents some challenges. A lot of it depends on the goals that we have for the patient.

Q: What do you recommend for primary [first] therapy to the prostate gland—surgery or radiation—in newly diagnosed patients with de novo oligometastatic disease extending beyond the pelvis?

Gershman: In my view, there still aren't sufficient data to recommend radical prostatectomy [surgical removal of the prostate gland] when there is evidence of cancer spread to other areas of the body. Studies investigating a role for it in this situation are going on now, and in time we might identify subsets of patients who could benefit from it. We do, however, have clinical trial data from the STAMPEDE study [full title: Systemic Therapy in Advancing or Metastatic Prostate

Curative therapy

Curative therapy entails aggressively treating all areas of cancer in the body, including the prostate itself, with a goal of eradicating the disease completely. Clinicians have traditionally avoided curative therapy for metastatic cancer. The thinking has been that aggressive treatments aren't justified because they have significant side effects and cures are unlikely. Metastatic cancer patients have generally been treated instead with palliative care, which consists of treating only symptoms, such as bone pain, trouble urinating, and neurological problems such as difficulty walking. This strategy has recently been called into question, as clinical trials increasingly show that multipronged treatments that include prostate-directed therapy improve survival in men with oligometastatic cancer. Whether radiation or surgery works better for treating the prostate in such a case is now a major area of investigation.

ROUNDTABLE DISCUSSION *continued*

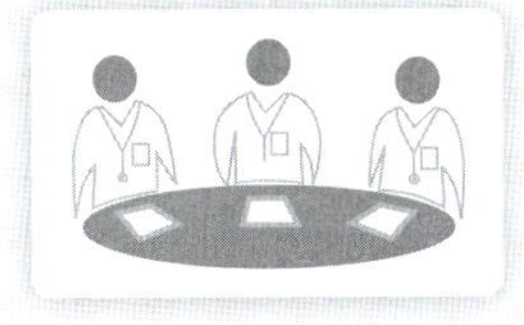

Cancer: Evaluation of Drug Efficiency] showing that radiation to the prostate extends survival.

Aghdam: I also favor radiation based on the STAMPEDE study, and would always prefer to give these prostate-directed treatments as part of a clinical trial.

Sternberg: Here at Weill Cornell, we're participating in a trial that randomizes men with oligometastatic disease to either radiation or radical prostatectomy. I find it a very hard trial to enroll patients into. They are not that eager. It's more difficult to enroll patients into this trial than to just offer them radiation therapy.

Einstein: I will say it is a hard sell for both patients and doctors to think about surgical removal of the prostate gland in the context of metastatic disease, because typically we really don't think of this being a situation where you're trying to achieve a cure. Given the recovery and side effects, we may need more data before doing surgery on these patients outside of clinical trials. I think the standard of care is increasingly ADT [hormonal therapy] including some of the newer agents such as abiraterone [Zytiga] or enzalutamide [Xtandi], and perhaps even chemotherapy as well. I think it's a little unclear from the existing clinical trial data if there's an added benefit from radiation in patients who get more modern systemic therapies. Patients have lot of options. We need to make sure they understand the uncertainties in the data, especially if they're entertaining the idea of doing something more aggressive than what we would have done traditionally.

Q:* *What about patients who have metastases in bones, but not in the pelvic lymph nodes? Do you still include the pelvic lymph nodes in your radiation field?

Aghdam: That's a really excellent question. And my answer is that if I don't see cancer in the lymph nodes, then I'm not going to treat them, given the side effects. My feeling is that if we are treating metastases, we should limit those treatments to what we can see with available imaging.

Sternberg: I would agree with that.

Q:* *Let's say you saw a 59-year-old patient with cancer in both sides of the prostate and three metastases in the bones. He's otherwise in great shape, and he wants to receive each and every therapy that offers a chance of a cure. He doesn't want to hear about the ongoing studies. He wants an answer from an expert. Would you radiate the patient? Would you give him a radical prostatectomy? What would you do with the oligometastases?

Gershman: I would counsel the patient that we, as yet, do not have convincing evidence that surgical removal of the prostate will provide a survival benefit, though it might prevent local symptomatic progression—meaning future issues that may cause problems or difficulties with urination. I would tell him the best setting for surgical removal of the prostate gland is in a clinical trial, and that there is currently evidence of benefits with radiation as primary therapy to the prostate. As data become available from ongoing trials, we will be able to determine whether surgery, as local therapy, may provide a survival benefit similar to radiation therapy. In addition, we will be better positioned to say who exactly is the best candidate for primary local therapy in oligometastatic disease. For the oligometastases to the bones, it would be reasonable to perform metastasis-directed therapy with radiation—that is, radiation targeting the sites that contain the metastases. The side effects are generally well tolerated and the treatments can reduce metastasis-related symptoms and potentially improve outcomes.

D'Amico: This is what I would say to the gentleman you've described: "I'm willing to treat your prostate because I know for sure this will delay recurrence of the cancer in the prostate gland and give you more time before you need additional follow-up therapy. This initial treatment will be radiation therapy to the prostate gland and systemic therapy, such as ADT, for at least two years. We may extend your longevity, but that I can't say for sure." Then I would add, "You have these three bone metastases. I'm willing to treat them as well with radiation and there could potentially be an additional benefit, but this is unknown."

Q:* *I recently consulted on a patient being treated at a prestigious West Coast academic institution. He's in his early 60s, his PSA was 16.4 ng/ml, he had Gleason 4+5 cancer on a prostate needle biopsy, several lymph nodes of less than a centimeter, negative bone and

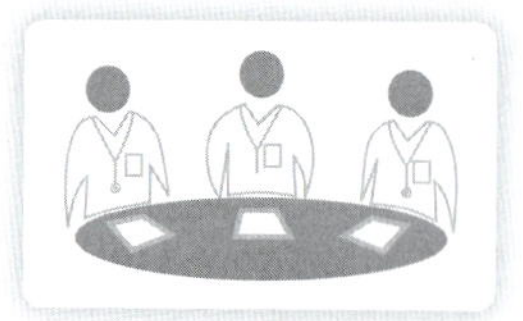

ROUNDTABLE DISCUSSION *continued*

CT scans, and no PET imaging. When he had radical prostatectomy, he had one positive lymph node and 12 negative lymph nodes. The PSA 46 months after surgery was undetectable. Shortly thereafter, it increased to 0.1, then 0.2, then 0.24 ng/mL. He then had hormonal therapy, but not radiation. What would you have recommended?

Sternberg: This is the kind of case where I would love to have PSMA PET, which can pick up metastases outside the pelvis when the PSA levels are still very low. Given that the patient had a high Gleason grade along with a positive lymph node, I would give radiation and 18 months of hormonal therapy.

Aghdam: I concur. The patient certainly has very high-risk disease. Hormonal therapy is absolutely appropriate and supported by evidence. I would treat the lymph nodes, and I would ask and defer to my medical oncology colleagues to determine the longest and most intense hormone therapy to give. If it was available, I would also want a PSMA scan to rule out any distant metastases.

D'Amico: We don't have very good evidence on the possible benefits of irradiating positive lymph nodes in postoperative patients. That said, my view is that if anybody with positive nodes is going to benefit from radiation, it's going to be someone with minimal pelvic disease and just one positive node. I would want further imaging to rule out metastases in bones or other areas that might have been missed. And I would want to check any positive findings with biopsies to confirm that metastases are indeed present.

Einstein: Given his Gleason score and the positive node that was already detected, I'd say there's a very high chance that other lymph nodes are involved. So, I agree on the need for advanced imaging, if possible, and think that certainly, at the very least, he should receive pelvic radiation plus ADT.

Q: When should hormonal, immune, or chemotherapies factor into the overall management of oligometastatic disease?

Sternberg: Hormonal therapies have in general been moved to earlier time points in treatment of patients with localized hormone-sensitive prostate cancer [cancer that has yet to be treated with hormonal therapies and which therefore has not yet had a chance to become resistant to hormonal therapy], as well as patients with oligometastatic cancer. Based on ambiguous clinical trial results with docetaxel [Taxotere], chemotherapy generally is not recommended for patients with oligometastatic cancer. And in general, immunotherapy has not been very effictive in treating prostate cancer, although we're hoping to change that.

Einstein: I agree the clinical trial evidence doesn't show a clear benefit from docetaxel. When it comes to ADT, the question is should we give it together with metastasis-directed therapy? Or should we give metastasis-directed therapy by itself to avoid or delay ADT or other systemic treatments? This is something we agonize a lot about with our patients. I would say the general practice is to give six months of ADT together with metastasis-directed therapy, but there is no optimal duration; some physicians go as long as 18 to 24 months. But sometimes we give the metastasis-directed treatments alone. And sometimes we use ADT with more intensive therapies like abiraterone. We really need a lot more research, and clinical trials are looking into metastasis-directed therapy with or without systemic treatments right now.

Q: Is it possible that SBRT itself might trigger immune reactions that lead to even broader and longer-lasting benefits?

Aghdam: Here you're talking about a potential "abscopal" effect, which means that radiation given to one part of the body somehow pushes the immune system to fight off cancer in unirradiated sites as well. We have seen evidence for abscopal effects in laboratory studies. And there is some clinical evidence of it in human patients, too. But there's also the possibility that radiation counteracts certain immune processes. So, I take a rather skeptical view of the abscopal effect when it comes to furthering survival in oligometastatic disease—at least as far as we understand it now.

Sternberg: There's been a lot written about the abscopal effect with radiation, but we still don't have good evidence for it with SBRT specifically.

Einstein: I would add that the patients who benefit most from metastasis-directed therapy appear to

ROUNDTABLE DISCUSSION *continued*

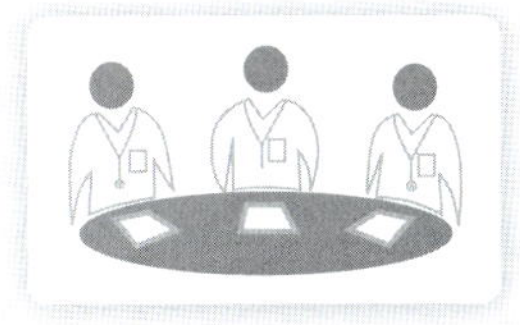

already have some anti-tumor T-cell activity [from the immune system] even before those treatments begin. It's possible that after immune cells start recognizing a cancer target, the addition of radiation somehow expands their activity, and helps to control the disease more effectively over the long term.

D'Amico: My view on this question is that an abscopal effect is theoretically possible. This is something that's being actively investigated.

Q: What are the appropriate endpoints to monitor when we're treating oligometastatic disease in clinical trials?

Sternberg: We can look at lowering PSA, but I would say that palliation [symptom control] of painful bones or even cure can be endpoints for small oligometastatic deposits.

Einstein: I think there are different bars, depending on how far along you are in your study. During an early exploratory study, you're often looking for quick, response-based outcomes. And in this case, changes in PSA are obvious to monitor, since increasing values suggest the cancer could be growing. The next level is a progression-free survival endpoint, such as how long it takes for tumors to start growing, or until the patient needs systemic therapy. The tallest order, of course, is overall survival, making people live longer over all, but we're also looking at quality of life. Hopefully we're allowing patients to live not just longer, but better.

Q: Now I want to go to the most important question. Do you think that previously incurable oligometastatic disease is curable with a multimodal approach that targets cancer from multiple angles?

D'Amico: If you biopsy an oligometastasis and find it has a mutation that you can target with currently available therapy, you're in a better position to go for a cure. You can treat the primary and any relevant nodal disease with radiation, and then use targeted therapy to eradicate any residual oligometastatic cancer. In my mind, this is the subgroup of patients who will benefit most from multimodal treatment.

Sternberg: Just to add to what Dr. D'Amico is saying, you could find a BRCA mutation, for instance, and then treat it with a type of targeted drug called a PARP inhibitor. Certainly, we need multimodality treatment. We need radiotherapy. We need surgery. We need to study the genomics and the genetics of our patients. And we need better agents than the ones we have now, because I don't know that we are curing patients, even though they are definitely living a lot longer than before.

Aghdam: The field is evolving such that we're shifting cancer progression further down the line. And we see the promise of systemic therapies that are going to revolutionize the management of these oligometastatic cancers. So, when I recommend local ablative therapy [therapy intended to completely eliminate the cancer, whether by surgery or radiation]—despite the limited supporting data and the side effects profile—my goal is for patients to lead a full life until the next excellent treatment comes along.

Einstein: I think that our more realistic hope is to prolong survival over all, and perhaps get some time off from cancer treatments, which is potentially really valuable as well. When you're managing a chronic disease, it's nice to have a break from treatment and the associated side effects. For some patients the first goal of metastasis-directed therapy is to delay the need for systemic treatments, which they may require for a long time. It's encouraging that prolonged remissions do occur in subsets of patients, and this suggests the chance of a cure.

Gershman: I will echo that. I think a cure in oligometastatic disease is likely a ways off. And meanwhile, there are other endpoints that are also highly relevant to patients, such as freedom from ADT. That's a reasonable patient-centered goal to accomplish realistically in the near term.

Q: Any parting comments?

Aghdam: This is an evolving field with many exciting developments, both in local and systemic therapies. I believe our ultimate goal is still to prolong overall survival, but we also need to consider what our patients value most—whether that's quality of life, managing side effects, or reducing burdens from systemic therapy. If we bring our patients into that conversation, then we can strategize on treatment with their best interests in mind.

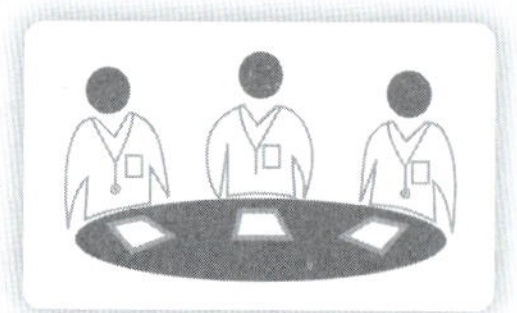

ROUNDTABLE DISCUSSION *continued*

Gershman: There's a large number of ongoing clinical trials investigating important issues in treatment, including treating the primary tumor in patients with de novo oligometastatic disease as well as treatments for oligorecurrent disease. And I think these studies are going to help us identify which patient populations stand to benefit most from various treatments.

Einstein: Oligometastatic disease is really an area that needs additional clinical research, and one in which we have the least well-defined standards of care. And that certainly calls for more and better trials that enroll as many patients as possible. We're having very nuanced discussions with patients about erring on the side of overtreatment versus undertreatment. I'm personally very excited about the potential for immune-based therapies, which need more testing. And we'd like to do better than simply committing patients to long-term hormone therapy, if we can go with other strategies first. So, this has been a great discussion, and thanks for having us.

Biomarkers and genetic testing

Aids to diagnosis and treatment

Biomarkers are molecular signatures of both normal and abnormal processes in the body. The National Institutes of Health defines them as substances that can be "objectively measured and evaluated as an indicator of normal biologic processes, pathogenic processes, or pharmacological responses to a therapeutic intervention."

Proteins, fragments of proteins, enzymes, DNA, and the RNA molecules that "read" DNA can all serve as biomarkers. Blood is an ideal source material because it's easy to collect and examine and contains some important biomarkers, but biomarkers can also be found in other body fluids, like saliva and urine, and in tissue itself. Biomarkers can inform decisions before, during, and after treatment.

More and better biomarkers are needed for many medical conditions but especially for prostate cancer. Too many screenings lead to biopsies that might have been avoided. Too many cancers are treated that didn't need to be treated because they weren't likely to cause any harm. For men who have prostate cancer and would benefit from treatment, a fuller menu of biomarkers could make it possible to tailor treatment to a man and his cancer so that the therapy is more effective.

With rapid advances in analytical methods, the number of biomarkers that have been identified for prostate cancer is growing steadily. More tests for measuring them are reaching the market, but head-to-head-comparisons of how these biomarkers perform in real-world settings are still needed to fully assess their potential for routine use.

One biomarker for prostate cancer screening has already been discussed at length in this report: prostate-specific antigen (PSA), a protein released by prostate tissue. The screening test measures levels of PSA in the blood. But the PSA test has two major problems. First, it's specific for the prostate but not for prostate cancer, so high levels may represent not cancer but benign prostatic hyperplasia (BPH) or some other problem related to the prostate. Second, even when high PSA levels predict prostate cancer correctly, the PSA test does not distinguish between aggressive cancers that need to be treated and indolent cancers that are growing so slowly they don't require treatment. Different ways of measuring PSA are beginning to solve these problems. They're discussed elsewhere in this report (see "Variations on the PSA test," page 48).

At the same time, doctors are turning to other biomarker tests to help them identify clinically significant prostate cancer, decide which men are appropriate candidates for active surveillance, and select treatment strategies. So far, only a few such assays have been commercially approved, and only a few studies have evaluated the short- and long-term consequences of using them in clinical decision making. However, it is an area of great promise.

Urine-based biomarkers

Eskra JN, Rabizadeh D, Pavlovich CP, et al. Approaches to Urinary Detection of Prostate Cancer. *Prostate Cancer and Prostatic Diseases* 2019;22(3):362–81. PMID: 30655600.

Margolis E, Brown G, Partin A, et al. Predicting High-Grade Prostate Cancer at Initial Biopsy: Clinical Performance of the ExoDx (EPI) Prostate Intelliscore Test in Three Independent Prospective Studies. *Prostate Cancer and Prostatic Diseases* 2021;Electronic publication ahead of print. PMID: 34593984.

Sanda MG, Feng Z, Howard DH, et al. Association Between Combined TMRPSS2:ERT and PCA3 RNA Urinary Testing and Detection of Aggressive Prostate Cancer. *JAMA Oncology* 2017;3(8):1085–93. PMID: 28520829.

Tosoian JJ, Trock BJ, Morgan TM, et al. Use of the MyProstateScore Test to Rule Out Clinically Significant Cancer: Validation of a Straightforward Clinical Testing Approach. *Journal of Urology* 2021;205(3):732–39. PMID: 33080150.

Van Neste L, Hendriks RJ, Dijkstra S, et al. Detection of High-Grade Prostate Cancer Using a Urinary Molecular Biomarker-Based Risk Score. *European Urology* 2016;70(5):740–48. PMID: 27108162.

Wysock JS, Becher E, Persily J, et al. Concordance and Performance of 4Kscore and SelectMDX for Informing Decision to Perform Prostate Cancer Biopsy and Detection of Prostate Cancer. *Urology* 2020;141:119–24. PMID: 32294481.

PubMed See page 120.

Urine-based biomarkers

Currently, the diagnosis of prostate cancer hinges on whether cancer cells are found in biopsy samples. But when PSA levels are only somewhat elevated—in the range of 4 to 10 ng/ml—about three out of every four biopsies come back negative. Urine-based tests are increasingly being used in these cases. If these tests rule out cancer, men can avoid unnecessary biopsies. In other cases, where the urine tests confirm cancer, test results are combined with information from biopsies so that doctors can better predict if a cancer is likely to spread.

Several urine tests have received FDA approval for their role in finding prostate cancer. While tissue biopsies are still the gold standard and urine tests provide only a limited range of information, in some cases it is information that otherwise cannot be obtained. (For references on the following examples, see "Urine-based biomarkers," at left.)

PCA3. When prostate cells become cancerous, their prostate cancer antigen 3 (PCA3) genes become overactive and produce telltale amounts of RNA molecules (molecules that deliver gene-specific instructions for making proteins) that leak into urine. Only prostate cancer cells overproduce PCA3 RNA, so unlike the PSA test, the PCA3 test is specific to cancer.

The FDA approved a commercially available PCA3 test called Progensa in 2012 for men ages 50 and older who have had one or more negative biopsies. The test is intended to help men and their doctors decide whether a repeat biopsy should be done. Evidence suggests the test is most accurate when PCA3 levels are either very low (signifying no cancer) or very high (signifying that cancer is present). According to Dr. Marc Garnick, editor in chief of the *Annual*, the usefulness of this test has been eclipsed by newer ones like SelectMDx (see "HOXC6/DLX1," page 99).

TMPRSS2:ERG gene fusion. When two genes—TMPRSS2 and ERG—switch places and fuse together, the result is known as the TMPRSS2:ERG fusion. This genetic rearrangement is found in about half of all prostate cancers, and measurable amounts of RNA from this fusion are present in urine. The TMPRSS2:ERG fusion is highly specific to prostate cancer—that's the good news. But because it's present in only half of prostate cancers, a lot of prostate cancers would be missed if it were the only biomarker used. Moreover, the fusion can't reliably distinguish low-grade from more aggressive cancers, and it doesn't predict how someone will respond to therapy. However, researchers reported in 2017 that combining TMPRSS2:ERG with PCA3 does improve its ability to detect more aggressive prostate tumors with a Gleason score of 7 or higher.

Two tests for this biomarker have become commercially available. Researchers at the University of Michigan developed a urine assay that combines PSA, PCA3, and TMPRSS2:ERG into a single value, called the MyProstateScore (MPS), which predicts the likelihood that a biopsy of a given tumor will show cancer. The assay was validated during a 2021 study of 1,525 men with suspected prostate cancer who had not yet had a biopsy. It detected high-grade cancer with better than 95% accuracy, and appears useful for ruling out unnecessary biopsies in men with negative results.

The other test, the ExoDx urinary prostate test, combines ERG with PCA3 and another marker called SPDEF in an assay designed to rule out prostate cancers with a Gleason score of 7 or higher. Pooled results from three validation studies reported in 2021 showed that 90% of the time, the test correctly identified men who did not have these high-grade tumors.

HOXC6/DLX1. Elevated levels of these two biomarkers can predict high-grade cancer in men flagged by PSA screening. Both biomarkers are messenger RNA (mRNA) molecules that carry genetic instructions for making proteins. SelectMDx is the brand name of a test that measures HOXC6 and DLX1 mRNA in urine, and it's used along with evaluations of prostate size, family history of prostate cancer, and DRE findings to assess the need for an initial biopsy in men with elevated PSA levels. A 2016 study with just over 900 men found the test could rule out high-grade cancers with a Gleason score of 7 or above with 98% accuracy, and potentially reduce unnecessary biopsies and overtreatment. However, in a study that was published in 2020, the assay did not perform as well as a combination of MRI and the 4Kscore (see page 49) when it came to accurately predicting clinically significant prostate cancers that were confirmed later with a biopsy. The National Comprehensive Cancer Network (NCCN) included the test in its 2019 guidelines for early prostate cancer detection. (For reference, see "Early detection guidelines," above right.)

Genetic and molecular tests of prostate tissue

Once a biopsy reveals cancer, a variety of different tests can be done to identify which genetic and other molecular biomarkers are present and active. Cancer is usually caused by genetic abnormalities, and doctors are now using increasingly sophisticated profiles of potentially affected genes and the proteins and metabolites they give rise to in order to distinguish between low- and intermediate-risk prostate cancers (which could be monitored with active surveillance) and more aggressive cancers (which should be treated more or less immediately). Importantly, expert guidelines have not yet provided definitive recommendations on how and when these tests should be used. Furthermore, data are still not available on how the use of these tests influences long-term outcomes. (For references on the various tests described here, see "Genetic and molecular biomarker research," at right.)

Panels of genes. The FDA-approved Prolaris test measures the RNA that "reads" the DNA of 46 genes involved in cell division and proliferation. Cells of aggressive prostate cancers divide more rapidly than those of low-risk prostate cancers, so the RNA levels that the Prolaris test measures should be higher if a cancer is likely to grow and spread. The test can be used at the time of diagnosis with a positive biopsy to determine whether a man's cancer falls into a low-, intermediate-, or high-risk category, and studies have shown it can predict the risk of dying from cancer and the risk that the disease may return and spread after initial treatment. This type of information can help doctors assess which men are suitable candidates for active surveillance. The evidence so far indicates that the Prolaris test is better at detecting aggressive cancers than it is at finding low-risk tumors that may not become life-threatening for many years. In 2017, Medicare expanded coverage of the test for use in men with intermedi-

Early detection guidelines

Mohler JL, Antonarakis ES, Armstrong AJ, et al. Prostate Cancer, Version 2.2019, NCCN Clinical Practice Guidelines in Oncology. *Journal of the National Comprehensive Cancer Network* 2019;17(5):479–505. PMID: 31085757.

Genetic and molecular biomarker research

Alam S, Tortora J, Staff I, et al. Prostate Cancer Genomics: Comparing Results from Three Molecular Assays. *Canadian Journal of Urology* 2019;26(3):9758–62. PMID: 31180305.

Armstrong AJ, Luo J, Nanus DM, et al. Prospective Multicenter Study of Circulating Tumor Cell AR-V7 and Taxane Versus Hormonal Treatment Outcomes in Metastatic Castration-Resistant Prostate Cancer. *JCO Precision Oncology* 2020;4:epub. PMID: 33154984.

Brooks MA, Thomas L, Magi-Galluzzi C, et al. GPS Assay Association with Long-Term Outcomes: Twenty-Year Risk of Distant Metastasis and Prostate Cancer–Specific Mortality. *JCO Precision Oncology* 2021;5:epub. PMID: 34036236.

Cedars BE, Washington SL 3rd, Cowan JE, et al. Stability of a 17-Gene Genomic Prostate Score in Serial Testing of Men on Active Surveillance of Early Stage Prostate Cancer. *Journal of Urology* 2019;6(6):381–87. PMID: 30958742.

Cullen J, Lynch JA, Klein EA, et al. Multicenter Comparison of 17-Gene Genomic Prostate Score as a Predictor of Outcomes in African American and Caucasian American Men with Clinically Localized Prostate Cancer. *Journal of Urology*;2021;205(4):1047–54. PMID: 33493001.

Fine ND, LaPolla F, Epstein M, et al. Genomic Classifiers for Treatment Selection in Newly Diagnosed Prostate Cancer. *BJU International* 2019;24(4):578–86. PMID: 31055874.

Graf RP, Hullings M, Barnett E, et al. Clinical Utility of the Nuclear-Localized AR-v7 Biomarker in Circulating Tumor Cells in Improving Physician Treatment Choice in Castration-Resistant Prostate Cancer. *European Urology* 2020;77(2):170–77. PMID: 31648903.

continued on page 100

ate-risk as well as low-risk prostate cancer. And in 2021, researchers presented results from a study showing that the test also helps to predict which men with unfavorable intermediate- or high-risk prostate cancer can safely avoid adding hormonal therapy to radiation. The researchers studied 741 patients who were given the test and then treated with either radiation therapy alone or in combination with hormonal therapy. Results showed that men with high test scores had a 21.2% risk of metastases at 10 years, compared with a 3.7% risk among those with low test scores.

Genomic Health's Oncotype DX test also analyzes gene activity by measuring RNA in tissue samples from a biopsy. Genomic Health started out with 727 candidate genes and winnowed down the list to 17 (plus five genes used for reference purposes) that its research showed were reliably associated with prostate cancer. Oncotype DX scores correlate with evidence of high-grade cancer, and scientists reported in 2019 that scores detected on the first biopsy tend to remain stable over time. This suggests that men on active surveillance might not need to have the test repeated on later biopsies. The test can also be used to determine the likelihood that a man's tumor is confined to the prostate, to ascertain the presence of high-grade cancer in tissues removed during surgery, and to estimate the likelihood of metastases or prostate cancer death within 10 years. In 2019, researchers reported that higher Oncotype DX scores were associated with more aggressive cancer and greater odds that PSA levels would increase in men who were treated with surgery after being on active surveillance. Studies published in 2020 and 2021 showed that Oncotype DX scores predict aggressive features in tumor biopsies equally well in Black and white American men. Also in 2021, researchers reported modeling results suggesting that Oncotype DX scores could predict the risk of metastases and prostate cancer death over 20 years of follow-up—an indication that the test provides helpful information on long-term outcomes. The results can help patients understand the potential risks and benefits of different treatment decisions. Oncotype DX is currently marketed for men with low- to intermediate-risk prostate cancer who may be trying to decide between active surveillance and more definitive treatment with surgery or radiation.

Another test, the Decipher prostate cancer test, looks at 22 genes involved in cancer cell proliferation, hormonal signaling, and tumor growth. The test was developed to help doctors determine if a surgically removed tumor has aggressive features and how quickly a man's cancer might metastasize. It's used mainly to make better-informed decisions about whether to proceed with more treatment, usually in the form of radiation after radical prostatectomy (surgery to remove the prostate). The Decipher test assigns a score from 0 to 1 for each biopsy sample, with scores above 0.6 predicting more aggressive cancer and the likelihood that a cancer will metastasize within five years if PSA levels rise again after surgical treatment. This information can help determine which patients would benefit from radiation therapy after radical prostatectomy. The test could also help some men avoid surgery by going on active surveillance if no aggressive features are found in their tumors. And a 2021 study with 352 patients and 13 years of follow-up suggests the test can also help doctors predict whether men with recurring prostate cancer will benefit from radiation.

Genetic and molecular biomarker research

continued from page 99

Guedes LB, Tosoian JJ, Hicks J, et al. PTEN Loss in Gleason Score 3 + 4 = 7 Prostate Biopsies Is Associated with Nonorgan Confined Disease at Radical Prostatectomy. *Journal of Urology* 2017;197(4):1054–59. PMID: 27693448.

Haney NM, Faisal FA, Lu J, et al. PTEN Loss with ERG Negative Status is Associated with Lethal Disease After Radical Prostatectomy. *Journal of Urology* 2020;203(2):344–50. PMID: 31502941.

Herelemann A, Huang HC, Alam R, et al. Decipher Identifies Men with Otherwise Clinically Favorable-Intermediate Risk Disease Who May Not Be Good Candidates for Active Surveillance. *Prostate Cancer and Prostatic Diseases* 2020;23(1):136–43. PMID: 31455846.

Kornberg Z, Cooperberg MR, Cowan JE, et al. A 17-Gene Genomic Prostate Score as Predictor of Adverse Pathology for Men on Active Surveillance. *Journal of Urology* 2019;202(4):702–09. PMID: 31026214.

Matuszczak M, Schalken JA, Salagierski M. Prostate Cancer Liquid Biopsy Biomarkers' Clinical Utility in Diagnosis and Prognosis. *Cancers* 2021;13(13):3373. PMID: 34282798.

Murphy AB, Carbanaru S, Nettey OS, et al. A 17-Gene Panel Genomic Prostate Score Has Similar Predictive Accuracy for Adverse Pathology at Radical Prostatectomy in African American and European American Men. *Urology* 2020;142:166–73. PMID: 32277993.

Scher HI, Graf RP, Schreiber NA, et al. Assessment of the Validity of Nuclear-Localized Androgen Receptor Splice Variant 7 in Circulating Tumor Cells as a Predictive Biomarker for Castration-Resistant Prostate Cancer. *JAMA Oncology* 2018;4(9):1179–86. PMID: 29955787.

Spratt DE, Yousefi K, Deheshi S, et al. Individual Patient-Level Meta-Analysis of the Performance of the Decipher Genomic Classifier in High-Risk Men After Prostatectomy to Predict Development of Metastatic Disease. *Journal of Clinical Oncology* 2017;35(18):1991–98. PMID: 28358655.

continued on page 101

Guidelines from the NCCN issued in 2018 and updated in 2020 state that men with favorable intermediate-risk prostate cancer (defined as Gleason 7, PSA levels of 10–20 ng/ml, and fewer than 50% positive biopsy cores) may consider results from the Decipher, Oncotype DX, Prolaris, and ProMark molecular assays (for more on ProMark, see "Protein-based tests," page 102) when deciding between active surveillance and treatment. Still, a 2019 study that compared results in 22 men who had at least two of the tests found the results didn't always agree. For patients who had both Decipher and Prolaris, for instance, results were in agreement only 67% of the time. The Prolaris results tended to favor active surveillance over surgery, while Oncotype DX favored the opposite approach. Dr. Garnick says the divergent findings reflect the need for more data on how treatment decisions based on molecular test results influence long-term outcomes.

PTEN. Loss of the PTEN gene is among the most common genetic changes that occur in prostate cancer, affecting roughly 40% of men who have the disease. PTEN is a tumor suppressor gene, so without it, the processes that keep cell division in check are missing, and cancer may develop. PTEN loss correlates with the hallmarks of aggressive prostate cancer, such as high Gleason scores, a shorter time to metastases, and recurrences relatively soon after surgery to remove the prostate, and a 2020 study showed the risks are greatest for men with ERG-negative tumors. By contrast, PTEN loss tends to be rare in men with low-risk prostate cancer, and in a 2019 study, researchers found that PTEN loss was frequently detected in biopsy samples from men whose cancers were worsening on active surveillance. Measuring PTEN in tissue isn't easy, so the test isn't typically performed, though with newer methods it could come into routine use.

AR-V7. The AR-V7 mutation affects a tumor cell's receptor for testosterone (the hormone that fuels prostate cancer growth). Scientists believe that mutated AR-V7 blocks hormonal treatments from binding with the receptor, the result being that the drugs have no effect. Men whose tumor cells test positive for the mutation tend to have worse responses to abiraterone (Zytiga) and enzalutamide (Xtandi) than men whose tumors test negative for the mutation. Doctors now test for the AR-V7 mutation to help predict if a man will respond to one of these two drugs. Those whose cells show the mutation might then receive chemotherapy instead. In fact, study results reported in 2018 showed that men with metastatic prostate cancer whose tumor cells tested positive for an AR-V7 mutation lived nearly twice as long on taxane chemotherapy as they did on enzalutamide (14.3 months compared with 7.3 months). The opposite was true in those whose tumor cells tested negative; they lived seven months longer on enzalutamide compared with taxanes. These results were validated in a 2019 study that enrolled 118 men with metastatic castration-resistant prostate cancer, of whom 10% or 24% were positive for AR-V7 (depending on the specific assay used to test for the mutation). Roughly half the men were treated with enzalutamide and the other half with abiraterone (five received both). Those who tested negative for AR-V7 lived nearly three times as long as those who tested positive for it.

Epigenetic changes. Mutations aren't the only factor that affects gene expression (how active a gene is). Chemicals that attach to DNA but leave the DNA sequence

Genetic and molecular biomarker research

continued from page 100

Tosoian JJ, Guedes LB, Morais CL, et al. PTEN Status Assessment in the Johns Hopkins Active Surveillance Cohort. *Prostate Cancer and Prostatic Diseases* 2019;22(1):176–81. PMID: 30279579.

Tward J, Lenz L, Flake DD, et al. The Clinical Cell-Cycle Risk (CCR) Score Is Associated with Metastasis After Radiation Therapy and Provides Guidance on When to Forgo Combined Androgen Deprivation Therapy with Dose-Escalated Radiation. *International Journal of Radiation Oncology, Biology, Physics* 2021;Electronic publication ahead of print. PMID: 34610388.

Wojno KJ, Costa FJ, Cornell RJ, et al. Reduced Rate of Repeated Prostate Biopsies Observed in Confirm MDx Clinical Utility Field Study. *American Health Drug Benefits* 2014;7(3):129–34. PMID: 4991397.

PubMed See page 120.

itself intact can also affect how active genes are. These changes, known as epigenetic changes, can be measured and used as biomarkers. Moreover, normal cells that are near cancer cells may also be affected. This "field effect" means that even if a biopsy is negative for cancer, it may contain cells with epigenetic changes that indicate that cancer is, in fact, lurking nearby in the gland.

ConfirmMDx is the brand name of a test that gives an epigenetic profile of three genes involved in the development of prostate cancer: GSTP1, APC, and RASSF1. Doctors use the test to rule out the possibility that prostate cancer may be going undetected in men with negative biopsy results. Uncertainty over these hidden cancers leads to high rates of repeat biopsies, along with the threat of infection and other complications, in men who are actually cancer-free. During a multicenter study in the United States, the test correctly identified men who did not have cancer with 88% accuracy. Five U.S. urology practices queried during that 2014 study reported that the test had allowed them to reduce the repeat biopsy rate to less than 5%. Applied nationwide, that figure would represent a substantial reduction from current practice. The test is approved for Medicare reimbursement.

Protein-based tests. The ProMark test measures eight proteins in cancerous prostate biopsy specimens that predict whether a cancer is likely to be aggressive or not. The test generates a score between 1 and 100, and as the score gets larger, so does the likelihood that a man has high-risk disease that could metastasize. The test was approved for Medicare coverage in 2016.

Blood-based tests

Like a urine test, a blood draw is much simpler to perform than a tissue biopsy and can yield some important information. This type of "liquid biopsy" is valuable for a couple of reasons. Cells and other material shed from tumors go into the blood before they reach urine or saliva. The presence of tumor cells in the blood is particularly interesting, as it indicates that cells have escaped from the primary tumor site and could seed new tumors elsewhere in the body. (For references on the following tests, see "Circulating tumor cells and DNA," at left.)

Circulating tumor cells. Cancer metastasizes when cells in the original tumor break away, get swept up into the bloodstream, and spread to other parts of the body. Researchers are developing ways to capture and measure those circulating tumor cells (CTCs) while they're en route. Capturing CTCs can reduce the need for follow-up biopsies of the prostate and other tissue and involves just a simple blood draw. Results can show whether a treatment is working. In fact, a 2018 study reported that a rising number of CTCs during the first 12 weeks of treatment was predictive for significantly worse survival in men being treated with abiraterone or chemotherapy.

Similarly, researchers reported in 2020 that they could detect CTCs in blood from 73 out of 203 patients who had undergone radical prostatectomy, even though they had undetectable PSA levels after the surgery. Importantly, circulating tumor cell detection was associated with a higher risk that PSA levels would later increase—a sign that the cancer may be returning.

Circulating tumor cells and DNA

Annala M, Vanderkerkhove G, Khalaf D, et al. Circulating Tumor DNA Genomics Correlate with Resistance to Abiraterone and Enzalutamide in Prostate Cancer. *Cancer Discovery* 2018;8(4):444–57. PMID: 29367197.

Armstrong AJ, Luo J, Nanus DM, et al. Prospective Multicenter Study of Circulating Tumor Cell AR-V7 and Taxane Vs Hormonal Treatment Outcomes in Metastatic Castration-Resistant Prostate Cancer. *JCO Precision Oncology* 2020. PMID: 33154984.

Campos-Fernández E, Barcelos LS, de Souza AG, et al. Research Landscape of Liquid Biopsies in Prostate Cancer. *American Journal of Cancer Research* 2019;9(7):1309–28. PMID: 31392072.

Goodall J, Mateo J, Yuan W, et al. Circulating Cell-Free DNA to Guide Prostate Cancer Treatment with PARP Inhibition. *Cancer Discovery* 2017;7(9):1006–17. PMID: 28450425.

Lorente D, Olmos D, Mateo J, et al. Circulating Tumour Cell Increase as a Biomarker of Disease Progression in Metastatic Castration-Resistant Prostate Cancer Patients with Low Baseline CTC Counts. *Annals of Oncology* 2018;29(7):1554–60. PMID: 29741566.

Murray NP, Reyes E, Fuentealba C, et al. Primary Circulating Prostate Cells Are Not Detected in Men with Low Grade Small Volume Prostate Cancer. *Journal of Oncology* 2014;2014:61274. PMID: 25210517.

Pak S, Suh YS, Lee DE. Association Between Postoperative Detection of Circulating Tumor Cells and Recurrence in Patients with Prostate Cancer. *Journal of Urology* 2020;203(6):1128–34. PMID: 31845840.

Torquato S, Pallavajjala A, Goldstein A, et al. Genetic Alterations Detected in Cell-Free DNA Are Associated with Enzalutamide and Abiraterone Resistance in Castration-Resistant Prostate Cancer. *JCO Precision Oncology* 2019;3:epub. PMID: 31131348.

PubMed See page 120.

One test for CTCs, called CellSearch, is already on the market, but researchers are trying to develop a more accurate test that costs less.

Aside from indicating the likelihood of a metastasis, any CTCs that are detected in a blood sample can be examined for a variety of mutations, such as AR-V7 (see page 101). A combined test for CTCs plus AR-V7 is available and is covered by Medicare.

Circulating tumor DNA. Prostate cancer cells can release their DNA into blood. This DNA is called circulating tumor DNA (ctDNA). It can supply useful clues about the nature of a man's cancer and how it's responding to treatment—and it's a lot more common in blood than CTCs themselves.

These are early days in the field, and much more validation is needed, but the initial evidence for ctDNA testing looks promising. For instance, in 2017, researchers reported that ctDNA can reveal newly acquired gene mutations that promote resistance to the drug olaparib (Lynparza), which is approved for men with advanced prostate cancer who test positive for inherited mutations affecting the BRCA1 and BRCA2 genes as well as mutations in another gene called ATM. Then in 2018, researchers reported that ctDNA test results predict if abiraterone or enzalutamide will work in patients with metastatic prostate cancer. About a third of patients who get these drugs don't respond to them. Results from the study showed that ctDNA in the nonresponders was typically positive for mutations in the drug's target—the androgen receptor. These results were validated in a 2019 study with 62 men that reached a similar conclusion.

In 2020, the FDA approved the Liquid CDx test, which analyzes 324 genes in ctDNA, including BRCA1, BRCA2, and ATM. The Liquid CDx test is now being used as a diagnostic tool to identify men with metastatic castration-resistant prostate cancer who are eligible for treatment with olaparib or another drug in the same class, rucaparib (Rubraca).

6

Erectile dysfunction and urinary incontinence

Solutions for some troublesome complications of prostate diseases

Erectile dysfunction (ED) and urinary incontinence are common side effects of prostate disease and its treatment. Surgical techniques such as nerve-sparing prostatectomy (in which the surgeon tries to avoid damaging the nerves that control function) and more precise radiation therapies have reduced but not eliminated them. However, treatments are available that may improve these conditions, if not cure them. See your urologist for an evaluation of the cause and severity of your condition and find out what he or she suggests. Most men can find a solution that will make the problem more manageable.

Treating erectile dysfunction

An erection begins when a touch, a look, or even a thought nudges the brain to send signals of arousal down the spinal cord and into the nerves of the penis. The nerves "talk" to one another by releasing nitric oxide and other chemical messengers, which boost the production of other important chemicals. These, in turn, initiate the erection by relaxing smooth muscle cells lining the tiny arteries that lead to the corpora cavernosa, side-by-side flexible cylinders that run the length of the penis (see Figure 11, below). As the arteries relax, the tissues swell with blood. The small veins that

Figure 11. What happens during an erection

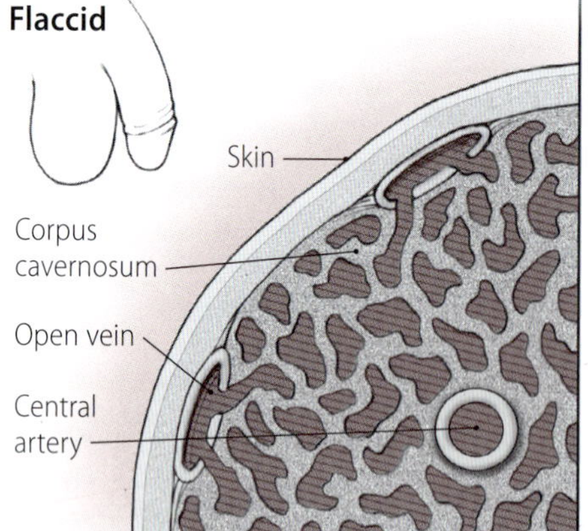

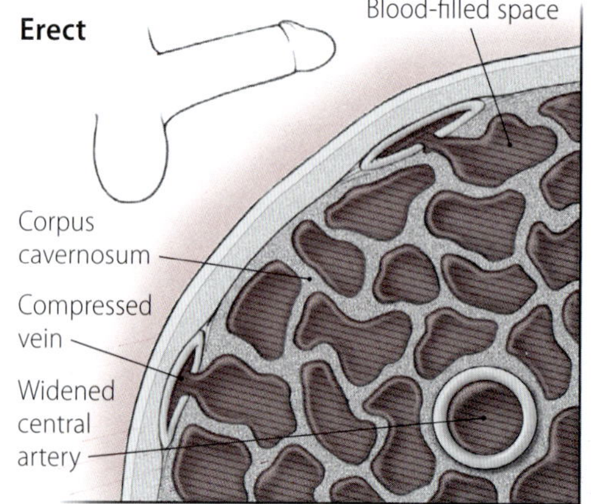

Chemical signals from the brain cause arteries in the penis to widen, allowing more blood to enter the erectile bodies known as the corpora cavernosa. These tissues swell with blood, causing an erection. At the same time, blood-engorged tissues compress the veins, keeping blood in the penis and maintaining the erection.

would normally allow blood to flow out of the penis are compressed, so the blood is trapped. The result is an erection.

Because the prostate is so closely intertwined with the other reproductive organs, any prostate-related problem or procedure has the potential of affecting sexual function. Some men experience short-term (generally less than one month) reductions in erectile function after a prostate biopsy, according to a 2021 review of 47 published papers. (For reference, see "Prostate biopsies and ED," at right.) Impairments can be more serious, however, once cancer is confirmed and treated.

Surgery for prostate cancer can sever some of the nerves and arteries that are necessary for an erection. Other nerves may be damaged and need time to heal. Only 10% to 23% of men below the age of 60 regain the degree of sexual potency they had before surgery, and the adoption of robotic methods has not brought a drop in long-term ED rates. Indeed, in a 2019 study, researchers studied ED rates in 2,364 men who had a radical prostatectomy (surgery to remove the prostate) for prostate cancer and found that there had been no improvements in recovery of erectile functioning during the prior decade, despite advances in surgical and postoperative care. But reported ED rates following prostate cancer surgery also vary widely, from a low of 14% to a high of 90%. The range is so wide as to be unhelpful for individual patients who would like to gauge their chances of developing erectile dysfunction after radical prostatectomy.

Radiation therapy for prostate cancer can also harm erectile tissues and the blood vessels that supply the penis and enable it to become erect. Erectile dysfunction is a side effect for roughly 40% to 50% of men treated with external beam radiation. And, in its advanced stages, prostate cancer itself can spread to the nerves and arteries necessary for an erection.

These are, though, just ranges and percentages. There's no reliable way to predict, at the individual level, who will develop ED after treatment and who will not. As you might expect, a man's age and health before treatment have a bearing on the chances. The data are complicated, but apart from a younger age and better overall health, such factors as lower prostate-specific antigen (PSA) levels, lower body mass index, and better sexual health and erectile function before surgery are associated with a lower risk of developing ED after radiation treatment. For men who have radical prostatectomy, age and body mass index are particularly important factors.

Other research has shown that men and their partners sometimes have unrealistic expectations about the ease with which men will regain erectile function after prostatectomy or radiation therapy. In men who do regain potency after surgery, recovery of function usually takes six to 12 months, even with nerve-sparing approaches and focal treatments that remove only cancerous portions of the prostate. For some, it takes a few years. Many men who have had a radical prostatectomy also have trouble achieving orgasm afterward, a problem that doesn't get discussed as often as it should (see "Orgasm after radical prostatectomy," page 106). (For references on ED associated with prostate cancer, see "ED following prostate cancer treatment," at right.)

Benign prostatic hyperplasia (BPH) is also a risk factor for ED, and some of the drugs used in treating it—notably dutasteride (Avodart) and finasteride (Proscar)—may cause ED as a side effect. Clinical trials suggest that finasteride causes ED in

Prostate biopsies and ED

Mehta A, Kim WC, Aswad KG, et al. Erectile Function Post Prostate Biopsy: A Systematic Review and Meta-Analysis. *Urology* 2021;155:1–8. PMID: 33524434.

ED following prostate cancer treatment

Capogrosso P, Vertosick EA, Benfante NE, et al. Are We Improving Erectile Function Recovery After Radical Prostatectomy? Analysis of Patients Treated Over the Last Decade. *European Urology* 2019;75(2):221–28. PMID: 30237021.

Donovan JL, Hamdy FC, Lane JA, et al. Patient-Reported Outcomes After Monitoring, Surgery, or Radiotherapy for Prostate Cancer. *New England Journal of Medicine* 2016;375(15):1425–37. PMID: 27626365.

Fallara G, Capogrosso P, Maggio P, et al. Erectile Function After Focal Therapy for Localized Prostate Cancer: A Systematic Review. *International Journal of Impotence Research* 2021;33(4):418–27. PMID: 32999435.

Favorito LA. Age and Body Mass Index: The Two Most Important Factors of Urinary and Erectile Function Recovery After Robot Assisted Radical Prostatectomy. *International Brazilian Journal of Urology* 2019;45(4):653–54. PMID: 31397985.

Schauer I, Keller E, Müller A, et al. Have Rates of Erectile Dysfunction Improved Within the Past 17 Years After Radical Prostatectomy? A Systematic Analysis of the Control Arms of Prospective Randomized Trials on Penile Rehabilitation. *Andrology* 2015;3(4):661–65. PMID: 26198796.

Smith ZL, Eggener SE. In Localised Prostate Cancer, Radical Prostatectomy Was Associated with More Sexual Dysfunction and Urinary Incontinence than Radiation or Active Surveillance. *Evidence-Based Medicine* 2017;22(5):192. PMID: 28814450.

PubMed See page 120.

Orgasm after radical prostatectomy

Although men are often most concerned that prostate cancer surgery will damage their erections, their orgasms also may suffer. Radical prostatectomy removes the seminal vesicles along with the prostate, leaving a man unable to ejaculate. Moreover, a small percentage of men—roughly 10%—can find orgasms painful after the surgery. Fortunately, that pain generally disappears within six months to a year. Orgasms may feel different after treatment, but they don't need to be less pleasurable or satisfying. Orgasm is also sensed in the brain, and this component can be just as intense as it was before surgery.

ED following BPH surgery

Soans J, Vazirian-Zadeh M, Kum F, et al. Can Surgical Treatment for Benign Prostatic Hyperplasia Improve Sexual Function? A Systematic Review. *Aging Male* 2020;23(5):770–9. PMID: 30955407.

Combination treatment for ED

Mykoniatis I, Pyrgidis N, Sokolakis I, et al. Assessment of Combination Therapies vs Monotherapy for Erectile Dysfunction: A Systematic Review and Meta-Analysis. *JAMA Network Open* 2021;4(2):e2036337. PMID: 33599772.

about 8% of men who take it and lowers libido in about 6%. In practice, however, doctors report that many more men experience these side effects (see "5-alpha-reductase inhibitors," page 27). Surgery and drugs used to treat BPH can also cause retrograde ejaculation, meaning semen flows back into the bladder instead of out of the penis during orgasm. However, a 2019 review of 16 studies reported no connections between surgical procedures for BPH and impotence. (For reference, see "ED following BPH surgery," below left.)

Many men are fearful or anxious about their first sexual experience after prostate disease treatment. As a result, they may avoid intimacy, touch, and sexual activity, and sexual partners may be reluctant to initiate any activity that could be perceived as pressuring. Many couples find it difficult to discuss their sexual relationship, but if they don't, the situation often gets worse. If a problem exists, researchers have found that the better a couple is at communicating with each other, the greater the chance they will achieve success through treatment.

You should see your doctor or another qualified health professional if you experience frequent or consistent ED after treatment for prostate disease. You may be asked to fill out a questionnaire about your erectile function, such as the International Index of Erectile Function, or IIEF (see Table 9, page 107), and answer questions about your sexual history, medical condition, and any medications that you take.

Next, your doctor may run tests to better understand what's happening physiologically. One such test is a nocturnal penile tumescence test, which monitors erections while you sleep, although this test is usually done in men whose ED is related to diabetes or heart disease rather than prostate cancer. During the test, a recording unit collects data on the number and duration of nocturnal erections, the change in the circumference of the penis, and penile rigidity. The measurements are made by two loops: one at the base of the penis and the other at the tip. Rigidity above 70% produces an erection suitable for penetration during sex; below 40% represents a flaccid penis. During eight hours of sleep, it's considered normal to have three to six erections lasting 10 to 15 minutes each, on average, though definitions of "normal" vary.

The remedies for ED resulting from prostate treatment are the same as those for ED from other causes (see Table 10, page 108). A treatment's effectiveness varies from individual to individual. According to a 2021 review, combinations of treatments for erectile dysfunction may work better for some men than a single treatment. (For reference, see "Combination treatment for ED," at left.) There may be some trial and error before you find one that works for you.

PDE5 inhibitors: Viagra and the other ED drugs

Avanafil (Stendra), sildenafil (Viagra), tadalafil (Cialis), and vardenafil (Levitra, Staxyn) belong to a class of drugs called PDE5 inhibitors. These drugs augment cyclic GMP, a chemical that relaxes smooth muscle in the penis, improving blood flow during sexual stimulation. They are easy to use and are effective for ED, helping 60% to 70% of men who take them. Success rates may be lower in men with diabetes, which can damage blood vessels.

Table 9. The Abridged International Index of Erectile Function (IIEF) questionnaire

The full-length IIEF questionnaire includes 15 questions to assess erectile function, orgasm ability, sexual desire, satisfaction with sexual intercourse, and overall satisfaction. An abridged version of the questionnaire with five questions, called the IIEF-5, focuses specifically on erectile function and satisfaction. A higher point total means better erectile function, and therefore less ED. Because the answers to some questions are subjective, clinicians also rely upon your medical history, a physical exam, and lab tests to diagnose and treat ED.

Rate your symptoms in the past six months:	1 point	2 points	3 points	4 points	5 points
How do you rate your confidence that you could get and keep an erection?	Very low	Low	Moderate	High	Very high
When you had erections with sexual stimulation, how often were your erections hard enough for penetration (entering your partner)?	Almost never or never	A few times (much less than half the time)	Sometimes (about half the time)	Most times (much more than half the time)	Almost always or always
During sexual intercourse, how often were you able to maintain your erection after you had penetrated (entered) your partner?	Almost never or never	A few times (much less than half the time)	Sometimes (about half the time)	Most times (much more than half the time)	Almost always or always
During sexual intercourse, how difficult was it to maintain your erection to completion of intercourse?	Extremely difficult	Very difficult	Difficult	Slightly difficult	Not difficult
When you attempted sexual intercourse, how often was it satisfactory for you?	Almost never or never	A few times (much less than half the time)	Sometimes (about half the time)	Most times (much more than half the time)	Almost always or always

Your score

Add up your points from each question

_____ + _____ + _____ + _____ + _____ = _____

What do the numbers mean?

5–7: severe ED
8–11: moderate ED
12–16: mild to moderate ED
17–21: mild ED
22–25: no ED

Sources: Rosen RC, Cappelleri JC, Smith MD, et al. Development and Evaluation of an Abridged, 5-Item Version of the International Index of Erectile Function (IIEF-5) as a Diagnostic Tool for Erectile Dysfunction. *International Journal of Impotence Research* 1999;11(6):319–26. PMID: 10637462.

Rosen RC, Riley A, Wagner G, et al. The International Index of Erectile Function (IIEF): A Multidimensional Scale for Assessment of Erectile Dysfunction. *Urology* 1997;49(6):822–30. PMID: 9187685.

PDE5 inhibitors can be used for ED related to prostate cancer treatment (both nerve-sparing radical prostatectomy and radiation therapy) and for ED related to BPH medications. Tadalafil is also approved as a treatment for BPH itself. But after a prostatectomy in which the nerve bundles could not be spared or were seriously damaged, the PDE5 inhibitors are ineffective and should not be taken.

Men are now routinely prescribed a PDE5 inhibitor immediately after nerve-sparing or partial nerve-sparing prostatectomy surgery in which the nerves were not too badly damaged. Small, daily doses of these drugs are thought to decrease the chances of developing ED by preserving smooth muscle function and oxygenation of tissues in the penis, and they may also help to limit or prevent what are usually minor reductions in penis size that can occur after surgery. A 2021 review of 22 studies comparing different penile rehabilitation strategies found that the PDE5 inhibitor sildenafil was especially helpful in regaining potency after prostate cancer surgery. (For reference, see "PDE5 inhibitors after prostate cancer surgery," at right.)

PDE5 inhibitors after prostate cancer surgery

Motlagh RS, Abufaraj M, Yang L, et al. Penile Rehabilitation Strategy After Nerve Sparing Radical Prostatectomy: A Systematic Review and Network Meta-Analysis of Randomized Trials. *Journal of Urology* 2021;205(4):1018–30. PMID: 33443457.

PubMed See page 120.

Table 10. Temporary treatments for erectile dysfunction

Treatment	How it works	How effective	How to use it
PDE5 inhibitors: avanafil (Stendra) sildenafil (Viagra) tadalafil (Cialis) vardenafil (Levitra, Staxyn)	These pills increase blood flow to the penis by augmenting cyclic GMP, a chemical that relaxes muscles in the penis, improving blood flow during sexual stimulation.	All these drugs have similar effectiveness (about 60% to 70%), but tadalafil lasts about 36 hours, whereas sildenafil and vardenafil last about eight hours, and avanafil lasts about six hours. Avanafil is the fastest acting, in about 15 to 30 minutes, whereas the others take 30 to 60 minutes.	In most cases, take a dose shortly before sexual activity. One low-dose tadalafil preparation can be taken daily instead of as needed. Don't take more than once in 24 hours. Do not take if you are also taking alpha blockers or nitrate medications.
Injections: alprostadil (Caverject, Edex)	The drug causes blood vessels to the penis to dilate, allowing engorgement with blood.	70% to 90% effective for all causes of erectile dysfunction. Most effective treatment for men whose erectile dysfunction results from prostate surgery.	Medicine is injected into the side of the penis. Erection occurs in five to 20 minutes and lasts 30 to 60 minutes. Shouldn't be used more than once in 24 hours.
Drug pellets: alprostadil (MUSE—medicated urethral system for erection)	Alprostadil, an injection therapy drug, is inserted into the penis in pellet form to open the blood vessels to the penis.	About 30% effective for all causes of erectile dysfunction.	An applicator, prefilled with alprostadil, is inserted into the tip of the penis. Erection begins in eight to 10 minutes and lasts for 30 to 60 minutes.
Vacuum pump	This noninvasive therapy is a pump that draws blood into the penis by creating a vacuum.	60% to 80% effective for all causes of erectile dysfunction.	The penis is placed in a plastic cylinder, then a vacuum is created with a manual or electric pump. When an erection occurs, a rubber ring is placed at the base of the penis to maintain the erection by preventing blood from escaping.

PDE5 inhibitors and cancer risk

Aoun F, Slaoui A, Walid AHO, et al. Association Between Phosphodiesterase Type 5 Inhibitors and Prostate Cancer: A Systematic Review. *Progrès en Urologie* 2018;28(12):560–66. PMID: 30201551.

Danley KT, Tan A, Catalona WJ, et al. The Association of Phosphodiesterase-5 Inhibitors with the Biochemical Recurrence–Free and Overall Survival of Patients with Prostate Cancer Following Radical Prostatectomy. *Urologic Oncology* 2021;Electronic publication ahead of print. PMID: 34284930.

Loeb S, Folkvaljon Y, Robinson D, et al. Phosphodiesterase Type 5 Inhibitor Use and Disease Recurrence After Prostate Cancer Treatment. *European Urology* 2016;70(5):824–28. PMID: 26743040.

PubMed See page 120.

One unconfirmed study suggested that PDE5 inhibitors may lead to an increase in PSA after surgery (a condition known as biochemical recurrence), suggesting the drugs might be driving cancer recurrence in some patients. But such claims have never been reproduced or substantiated and should not preclude the use of these agents in men who have had a radical prostatectomy. Indeed, a large study published in 2021 generated precisely the opposite finding. Researchers studied 3,100 men who underwent a radical prostatectomy between 2003 and 2015, split between those who used PDE5 inhibitors and those who did not. After 10 years, 93.2% of the men who had used PDE5 inhibitors were still free of biochemical recurrence, compared with 85.3% of those who hadn't used the drugs. (For references, see "PDE5 inhibitors and cancer risk," at left.)

PDE5 inhibitors are unlikely to produce an erection during the first six months or so after surgery, so men have to be patient. The delay is fortunate, because an erection too soon after surgery could cause surgical stitches that hold tissues together to break open, causing bleeding.

Costs for sildenafil and tadalafil have dropped sharply since generic versions of the drugs came on the market in 2017 and 2018, respectively. Other PDE5 inhibitors remain expensive, and some health insurance plans don't cover them or cover just a few pills per month, although men can get discount coupons from manufacturers. Your pharmacist may also be able to check for coupons that will save you money (generally about 10% lower than retail). Medicare generally doesn't pay for medications used in treating ED, although some Medicare Part D plans cover generic versions. Tadalafil —the only PDE5 inhibitor that also has FDA approval for treating BPH—may be covered if prescribed for that purpose. Check with your plan to be sure.

The drugs shouldn't be taken more than once a day, and you shouldn't take them if you are also taking nitroglycerin or another nitrate drug for heart disease. Men who take certain alpha blockers that tend to lower blood pressure also need to exercise caution; in fact, all men with heart disease should be careful because PDE5 inhibitors tend to lower blood pressure. If you take a PDE5 inhibitor and wind up going to the hospital with heart attack symptoms, be sure to tell the medical personnel there that you have taken one of these ED drugs.

Short-term side effects of PDE5 inhibitors include headache, flushing, upset stomach, and nasal congestion. Temporary disturbances in vision have been reported. Some men experience a bluish tinge to their sight. Vision loss and hearing loss are rare. Another possible though relatively rare complication is priapism, an erection that lasts too long. Any man who has an erection for more than four hours should go to the emergency room to receive a counteracting drug. Prolonged erections can cause permanent impotence because of damage to penile tissues, perhaps related to ischemia (inadequate blood supply).

Injectable drugs

The idea of injecting a drug into the penis is upsetting at first. But for men who can't take a PDE5 inhibitor because of its side effects or for some other reason, or who don't respond to PDE5 inhibitors, injectable drugs are a good alternative (see Figure 12, below). Moreover, injection therapy is often more effective than PDE5 inhibitors for men whose ED is related to radical prostatectomy, because the injected drug goes directly into the blood vessels that control erections. When you take a pill, the drug

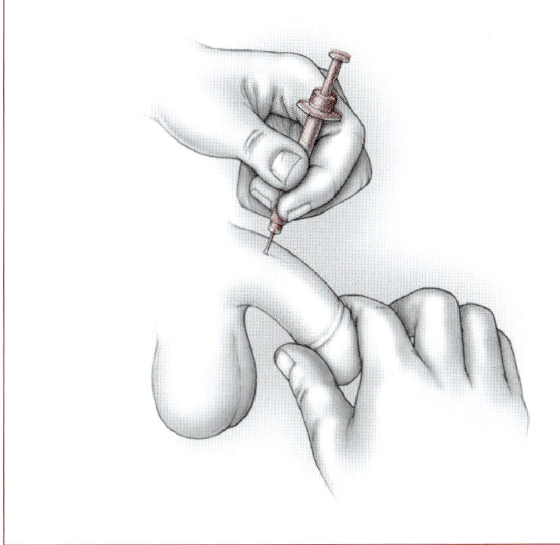

Figure 12. Injection therapy

Using a small needle, a man can inject one or more prescription drugs into the side of his penis. The injected drugs work by relaxing the smooth muscle tissue of the penis and allowing blood to flow into the erectile tissue to produce an erection. However, they can also cause priapism (an erection that can last for hours in the absence of stimulation), which is a medical emergency.

Injection therapy for ED

Bearelly P, Phillips E, Pan S, et al. Long-Term Intracavernosal Injection Therapy: Treatment Efficacy and Patient Satisfaction. *International Journal of Impotence Research* 2020;32(3):345–51. PMID: 31477852.

Misrha K, Loeb A, Bukavina L, et al. Management of Priapism: A Contemporary Review. *Sexual Medicine Reviews* 2020;8(1):131–39. PMID: 30898593.

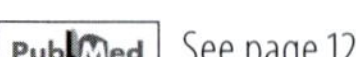
See page 120.

has to be metabolized and may not reach the target tissue in high enough concentrations to be effective. A 2020 study showed that injectable treatments were safe and effective in 105 men who had been using them for more than eight years on average. The main side effects are mild to moderate pain, bruising, or scarring. In some cases, they cause priapism (an erection that can last for hours in the absence of stimulation), which is a medical emergency that may require letting some blood out of the penis to enable the penis to relax and not stay erect. (For references, see "Injection therapy for ED," at left.)

In the United States, the only injectable drug specifically approved for ED is alprostadil (Caverject, Edex). Alprostadil (prostaglandin E1) is a potent vasodilator, meaning it widens arteries, allowing them to carry more blood. Other drugs used for injectable therapy for ED include papaverine, another vasodilator, and phentolamine, an alpha blocker. Those two drugs are sometimes combined with alprostadil in a three-part mixture. Meanwhile, experimental agents are being investigated.

Urethral suppositories

As an alternative to injection, alprostadil is also available as tiny pellets that can be inserted into the penis shortly before intercourse. These pellets are part of a therapy called the medicated urethral system for erection (MUSE).

This therapy involves inserting a pellet about an inch into the penis, using a disposable plastic applicator. From there, the surrounding tissue quickly absorbs the drug. Some men find MUSE easier to use than injections, but about 10% of men who try it find the application mildly painful, and about 3% become dizzy and develop low blood pressure. Men should not use MUSE more than twice in 24 hours.

Vacuum pump

Until prescription medications came along, the only proven at-home therapy for ED involved using a vacuum pump. With this therapy, you lubricate your penis and put it into an airtight plastic cylinder that's attached to a handheld or battery-operated pump that creates a vacuum (see Figure 13, page 111). The negative pressure draws blood into the corpora cavernosa, the columns of spongy tissue that fill with blood to produce an erection. Once an erection occurs, which usually takes about five minutes, you remove your penis from the cylinder and fit an elastic band around the base of the penis to prevent blood from draining away. The erection lasts until the band is removed.

Vacuum pumps are noninvasive and highly effective when used correctly, working for about 80% of men. Their advantage over medication is that they can be used as often as a man wants. Men who have intercourse only occasionally may find a vacuum pump satisfactory. There are several disadvantages. The pumps require a bit of manual dexterity, and having to fuss with the device can interrupt lovemaking. In addition, the erection doesn't feel as natural as one produced by a drug; although firm, it can be somewhat floppy because it does not extend down into the base of the penis. About 10% of men have side effects, such as pain, bruising, or difficulty ejaculating, any of which can cause discomfort during sexual activity. Dr. Marc Garnick, editor in chief

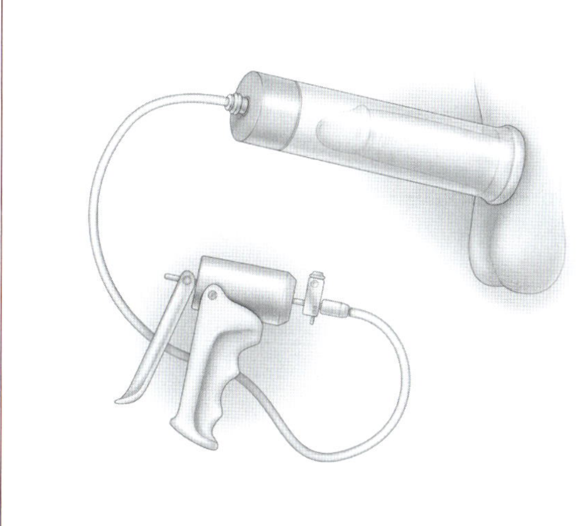

Figure 13. Vacuum pump

To achieve an erection, a man puts his lubricated penis into an airtight plastic cylinder attached to a handheld or battery-operated pump. Pumping air out of the cylinder creates a vacuum, which increases blood flow to the penis and causes an erection. An elastic band placed at the base of the penis maintains the erection.

of the *Annual*, cautions that men should be instructed in the proper use of a vacuum pump, and that in his experience, men who use it too soon after prostate cancer surgery can pull their stitches out of place.

Penile implants

Penile implants are a possibility for men who have tried ED medications and vacuum pumps with no success. Men with penile implants can have an erection at any time—and maintain it for as long as they want—allowing for great spontaneity. There are two basic varieties:

Inflatable implants. These may have a two- or three-piece design. Three-piece implants consist of a fluid-filled reservoir in the abdomen, a pump with a release valve in the scrotum, and two inflatable cylinders in the penis. Squeezing the pump transfers fluid from the reservoir into the cylinders, causing an erection. Pushing the release valve drains the fluid back into the abdominal reservoir. In two-piece implants, fluid-filled reservoirs are in the rear portion of the cylinders; the pump is in the scrotum. Bending the penis returns the fluid to the reservoir.

The devices have evolved over time, and there has been substantial progress with respect to function, ease of use, and reductions in postoperative complications and pain. According to a 2018 study focused on use in New York State, the trend is increasingly moving in favor of inflatable implants over other varieties, and a report published in 2019 found that inflatable implants were associated with greater satisfaction scores at one year. One drawback to inflatable implants, however, is the risk of mechanical trouble, such as a leaky reservoir that requires surgical repair, although most devices are fairly durable and last 10 years or longer. Another is the possibility that the penis will get shorter, although a variety of recent techniques to increase penile length in men who undergo the procedure have improved patient satisfaction.

Semirigid, or malleable, rods. As the name implies, this type of implant consists of bendable rods, usually constructed of braided stainless steel wires or articulating plastic discs, covered with silicone. The rods are bent upward to have sex and pointed down to conceal the penis under clothing.

Most patients choose an inflatable device because the penis looks more natural than with semirigid rods. Malleable devices have their pros and cons, too. They are easier to manipulate than inflatable implants, and a single incision makes them simpler to insert surgically. But because the rods always remain firm, their presence is harder to conceal. (For a more detailed comparison, see Figure 14, page 113.)

Regardless of the model chosen, patients and their partners report a high overall degree of satisfaction with penile implants. Of 425 men in a British study of penile implants, most of whom had the malleable variety, 89% could have sexual intercourse, and 81% were satisfied with the implant results. Similar results were achieved in a study of 149 patients who were given three-piece inflatable implants. Published in 2019, that study found that nearly half the implants were still working properly after an average of 17 years. Among men who continued to use the devices during that period, most reported being highly satisfied with them. Still, patients need to consider penile implant surgery carefully. The infection rate is the same as it is for other surgical procedures—about 1% to 3%, though the rates are also falling as surgical techniques improve and the use of antimicrobial coatings gains in popularity, according to a 2020 review study. (For references, see "Penile implants," at left.)

The procedure to implant a penile device takes about one to two hours. Strenuous physical activities should be avoided for about a month; sexual activity can resume in four to six weeks.

Patients and their partners are generally more satisfied with the results if they know what to expect from a penile implant. If possible, you and your partner should meet with the doctor together before surgery. Make sure you understand the risks and benefits of the procedure and how the device works.

Treating urinary incontinence

The involuntary leakage of urine is another common and embarrassing side effect of prostate disease and its treatment, and it is generally the most dreaded and unwelcome of all potential side effects from prostate cancer treatment—even more than erectile dysfunction. For men who have had a prostatectomy, urine leakage is a frequent side effect, particularly for men with large prostates, but one that often subsides gradually over the first two years following surgery. Even men who are still incontinent a year after radical prostatectomy can experience incremental improvements. A 2019 study of 322 men who had a radical prostatectomy for localized prostate cancer found that 58% regained good urinary functioning within three months, and just over 91% regained it within two years. (For references to research mentioned throughout this section, see "Urinary incontinence," page 114.) Although irritation, burning, and painful urination are the most common urinary side effects of radiation therapy, incontinence—though uncommon with a highly skilled radiation oncologist—can also occur.

If you experience urinary problems following prostate treatment, your doctor may recommend a urodynamic evaluation—a diagnostic session to help determine the

continued on page 114

Penile implants

Akakpo W, Pineda MA, Burnett AL. Critical Analysis of Satisfaction Assessment After Penile Prosthesis Surgery. *Sexual Medicine Reviews* 2017;5(2):244–51. PMID: 28143706.

Capogrosso P, Pescatori E, Careceni E, et al. Satisfaction Rate at 1-Year Follow-Up in Patients Treated with Penile Implants: Data from the Multicentre Prospective Registry INSIST-ED. *BJU International* 2019;123(2):360–66. PMID: 29956870.

Castiglione F, Ralph DJ, Muneer A. Surgical Techniques for Managing Post-Prostatectomy Erectile Dysfunction. *Current Urology Reports* 2017;18(11):90. PMID: 28965315.

Chierigo F, Capogrosso P, Deho F. Long-Term Follow-up After Penile Prosthesis Implantation: Survival and Quality of Life Outcomes. *Journal of Sexual Medicine* 2019;16(11):1827–33. PMID: 31501062.

Dinerman BF, Telis L, Eid JF. New Advancements in Inflatable Penile Prosthesis. *Sexual Medicine Reviews* 2021;9(3):507–14. PMID: 33610493.

Kashanian JA, Golan R, Sun T, et al. Trends in Penile Prosthetics: Influence of Patient Demographics, Surgeon Volume, and Hospital Volume on Type of Penile Prosthesis Inserted in New York State. *Journal of Sexual Medicine* 2018;15(2):245–50. PMID: 29292061.

Mahon J, Dornbier R, Wegrzyn G, et al. Infectious Adverse Events Following the Placement of a Penile Prosthesis: A Systematic Review. *Sexual Medicine Reviews* 2020;8(2):348–54. PMID: 31519461.

Minervini A, Ralph DJ, Pryor JP. Outcome of Penile Prosthesis Implantation for Treating Erectile Dysfunction: Experience with 504 Procedures. *BJU International* 2006;97(1):129–33. PMID: 16336342.

Shah BB, Kent M, Valenzuela R. Advanced Penile Length Restoration Techniques to Optimize Penile Prosthesis Placement Outcomes. *Sexual Medicine Reviews* 2021;9(4):641–49. PMID: 32653404.

PubMed See page 120.

Figure 14. Penile implants compared

Three-piece inflatable implant

Advantage

- Acts and feels more like a natural erection than semirigid models.

Disadvantages

- Requires more manual dexterity than other implants.
- Possibility of leakage or malfunction.
- Most expensive type of implant.
- Requires the most extensive surgery of all implants.

Comments

- The inflate/deflate device is implanted in the scrotum. Squeeze pump to inflate, and press the release valve to deflate.
- The fluid reservoir is implanted in the abdomen.
- Lock-out valve can prevent unintended inflation.

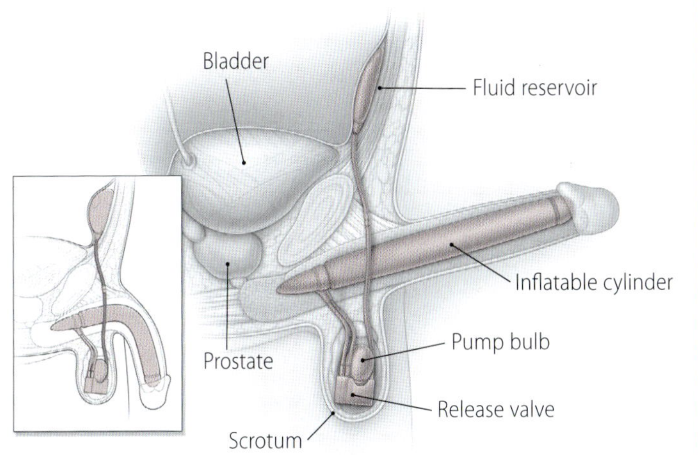

Two-piece inflatable implant

Advantages

- Penis looks more natural in erect and flaccid states than with the semirigid implant.
- Easier to operate than the three-piece implant.
- No abdominal incision.

Disadvantage

- Possibility of leakage or malfunction.

Comments

- Squeeze and release the pump several times to move fluid into the penile cylinders. Bending and holding the penis causes the cylinders to soften.
- The penis does not deflate as fully as with the three-piece implant.

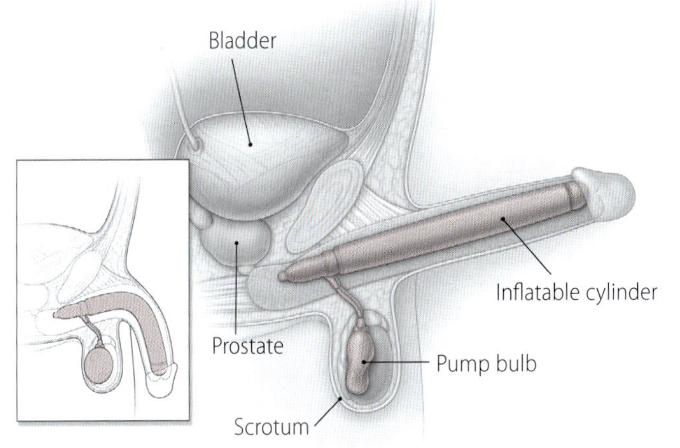

Semirigid (malleable) implant

Advantages

- Easy to use, especially for those with limited dexterity.
- Requires the least extensive surgery.
- Fewest parts, so less chance of malfunction.
- Least expensive type of implant.

Disadvantages

- Constantly firm.
- Somewhat harder to conceal than inflatable implants, but new designs make this less of a concern than in the past.

Comment

- For intercourse, lift the penis and make the rods as straight as possible.

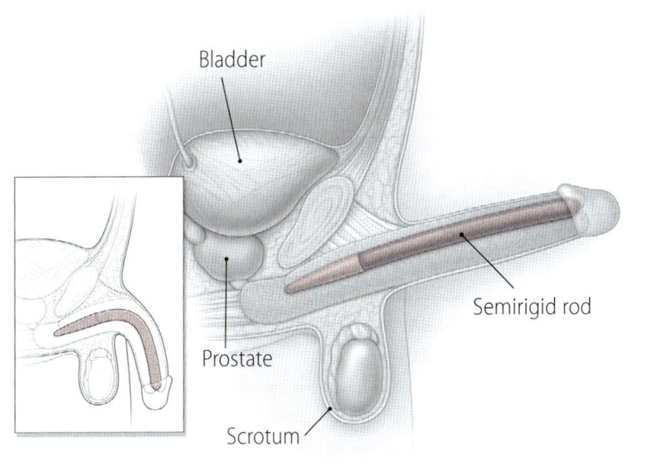

continued from page 112

nerve and muscle function of your bladder and urethral sphincter (the ringlike muscle that controls urine flow). This will help pinpoint the exact nature of the problem.

Before seeing your doctor, keep a written record of your urination habits for at least three days. Note when the leaking occurred, what you were doing at the time, what appears to make the problem worse, and what appears to make the problem better. This will help your doctor determine the type or types of incontinence you have.

Three types of incontinence and frontline treatments

There are three main types of urinary incontinence that may develop after treatment for prostate cancer. Treatment varies according to type.

Stress incontinence. This type of incontinence is characterized by the leakage of small amounts of urine when you cough, sneeze, lift a heavy object, exercise, or otherwise put pressure on your bladder. One cause of stress incontinence is damage to the external urethral sphincter, a band of muscle tissue that controls "downstream" urine flow from the bladder and through the urethra. Surgery on the prostate, such as transurethral resection of the prostate (TURP) or prostatectomy, can cause such damage.

For stress incontinence, pelvic muscle exercises and biofeedback training so you can control those muscles can help you sense your bladder filling, allowing you to delay voiding until you reach a toilet. The pelvic floor comprises the group of muscles connected to the pubic bone in the front and the tailbone, or coccyx, in the back. Pelvic floor exercises—also known as Kegel exercises (below left)—can help with urinary incontinence after radical prostatectomy for prostate cancer. Some research has found that pelvic floor exercises could have the added bonus of helping with ED after prostatectomy. Also, electrodes placed on the skin or in a probe inserted in the anus can be used to electrically stimulate pelvic muscles and possibly strengthen them. Research shows some short-term benefits to this approach but is silent on whether it lasts.

Bulking agents, which have been used extensively in men who have undergone radical prostatectomy, are another option. The most commonly used bulking agent is collagen, the protein that gives skin its tone. (Plastic surgeons use collagen as a filler in cosmetic procedures.) In an outpatient procedure, a physician injects the bulking agent into the area once occupied by the prostate to support the urethral muscles, so the patient doesn't lose urine as easily. However, any success at regaining continence with bulking agents tends to diminish within a few months because the body absorbs the material. Still, as a temporary measure, this is a viable option for men who cannot undergo invasive surgery.

Urge incontinence. Urge incontinence occurs when the bladder develops a spasm. It suddenly contracts and expels urine. BPH seems to leave the bladder prone to such irritation.

Some people with urge incontinence find that retraining the bladder is effective. This technique involves increasing the storage capacity of the bladder by learning to suppress sudden urges to urinate and by prolonging the interval between urinations.

The most effective drugs for urge incontinence are oxybutynin (Ditropan), tolterodine (Detrol), and some of the tricyclic antidepressants. For incontinence that

Urinary incontinence

Das AK, Kucherov V, Glick L, et al. Male Urinary Incontinence After Prostate Disease Treatment. *Canadian Journal of Urology* 2020;27(S3):36–48. PMID: 32876001.

Radadia KD, Farber NJ, Shinder B, et al. Management of Postradical Prostatectomy Urinary Incontinence: A Review. *Urology* 2018;113:13–19. PMID: 29031841.

Rajih E, Meskawi M, Alenizi AM, et al. Perioperative Predictors for Post-Prostatectomy Urinary Incontinence in Prostate Cancer Patients Following Robotic-Assisted Radical Prostatectomy: Long-Term Results of a Canadian Prospective Cohort. *Canadian Urological Association Journal* 2019;13(5):E125–31. PMID: 30332593.

PubMed See page 120.

Kegel exercises

The strength and proper action of your pelvic floor muscles are important in maintaining continence. Here's how to do basic pelvic muscle exercises, named for Arnold Kegel, the physician who first developed them:

1. Pretend you are trying to avoid passing gas. You will feel a contraction more in the back than in the front, as if you are pulling the anal area in.
2. Practice both short contractions and releases and longer ones, gradually increasing the strength of the contraction and holding it for up to 10 seconds.
3. Repeat multiple times, several times a day.

results from treatments for prostate enlargement—such as TURP, which may produce bladder instability and urge incontinence—anticholinergic drugs such as propantheline (Pro-Banthine) and dicyclomine (Bentyl) may help.

Overflow incontinence. Overflow incontinence is the result of partial obstruction, such as an enlarged prostate. Because the bladder cannot empty completely, it becomes overfilled or distended, and urine dribbles from the urethra. It can also occur when the bladder muscle becomes severely weakened—a problem that can develop as a result of BPH if the bladder muscle becomes thick from straining to urinate.

Alpha blockers—such as alfuzosin (Uroxatral) and tamsulosin (Flomax)—may improve overflow incontinence caused by BPH. These drugs help relax urethral muscles, decreasing urinary retention and the tendency to leak urine.

Options for severe incontinence

For more severe incontinence, there are several surgical procedures that can be performed to achieve dryness.

Artificial urinary sphincter. The leading therapy for severe incontinence after prostate cancer surgery is the surgical placement of an artificial urinary sphincter (see Figure 15, below). The procedure involves placing a small, fluid-filled inflatable

Figure 15. Artificial urinary sphincter

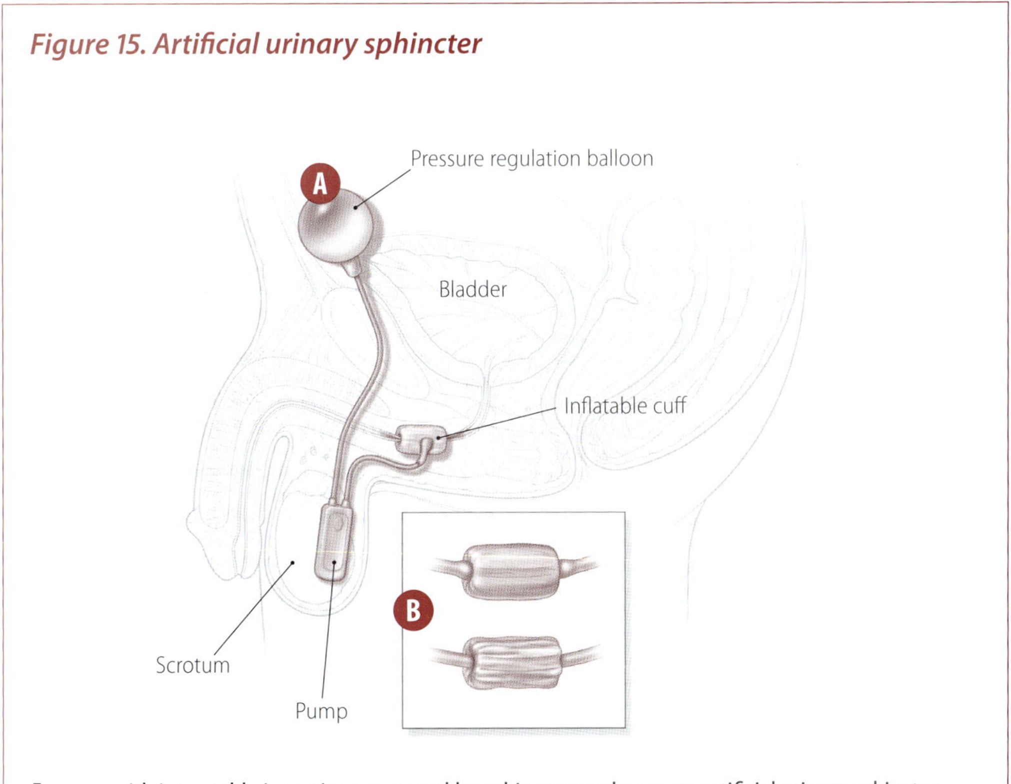

For men with intractable incontinence caused by sphincter weakness, an artificial urinary sphincter is a possible solution. After it is surgically inserted, the fluid-filled cuff compresses the urethra to stop the flow of urine (**A**). To allow urination, a man squeezes a small pump, which deflates the cuff enough so that urine can pass (**B**). The cuff automatically refills.

cuff around the urethra and a small pump in the scrotum. When it's inflated, the cuff squeezes the urethra so urine can't flow through it. When a man is ready to urinate, he squeezes the pump, which deflates the cuff enough so that urine can flow. When he is finished, the cuff then reinflates on its own.

Success rates for artificial sphincter surgery are relatively high. Continence isn't restored immediately, however. It may take four to six weeks to heal from the surgery, during which time the pump cannot be activated. Men who undergo this procedure may also experience complications such as infection, erosion of tissue around the implants, and device malfunction, which may require additional surgery.

Living with urinary incontinence

Even if your urinary incontinence can't be cured, it can be managed. In addition to the treatments already described, absorbent underclothing is available that's no more bulky than normal underwear and can be worn easily under everyday clothing. Highly absorbent disposable pads are available in drugstores.

In another approach, a flexible tube (called an indwelling catheter) can be placed in the urethra to collect urine in a container. However, long-term catheterization, although sometimes necessary, can create many problems, including urinary infections. When a long-term catheter is necessary, one option to consider is a suprapubic catheter that is inserted through the abdomen and then into the bladder. Finally, an external collecting device is another option. This condom-like device is fitted over the penis and connected to a drainage bag. It can be removed as necessary.

Coping with incontinence can be frustrating, especially if the first few treatments you try don't yield the results you're seeking. But the good news is that there are many choices for managing incontinence. Through trial and error, you may be able to find an option that works well for you. Just remember that this process can take time, so you'll probably need to exercise some patience.

Take charge of your condition

A brief review of changes that may improve your health

Coping with prostate disease isn't easy. If you have prostatitis, you may find that established treatments aren't particularly effective. You may become frustrated if medications for benign prostatic hyperplasia (BPH) don't alleviate the frequent urge to urinate. Prostate cancer treatment can be a long haul. You can, however, take steps to meet these challenges. This chapter offers some suggestions.

Participate in a clinical trial

Doctors often suggest that patients take part in clinical trials to gain access to promising treatments and medications. Clinical trials drive medical progress, especially in cancer. But your decision to enroll should be an informed one. Make sure you know why the study is being done, who is paying for it, what the experimental therapy entails, and how it affects other aspects of your treatment. Also, you should realize that there is a good chance you will be randomly assigned to standard therapy or even a placebo rather than the experimental treatment, because clinical trials require a control group for the sake of comparison, to see if the new treatment delivers better results.

Join a support group

Some doctors suggest that patients attend a support group. Even if you don't feel the need for emotional support, these groups can be a great source of information. To find a group in your area that deals with your condition, ask your doctor or check with your hospital. You can also find support groups through Zero—The End to Prostate Cancer, at https://zerocancer.org.

Make smart lifestyle changes

Many of the same lifestyle changes that have been shown to help with overall health can improve quality of life for men with prostate disorders—and may help prevent prostate cancer from recurring (secondary prevention). A number of observational studies indicate that a healthy diet, exercise, weight control, and smoking cessation may all help. (For reference, see "Secondary prevention," at right.)

Diet

Good nutrition is important for everyone, but it is especially a concern for men with prostate cancer. "Should I change my diet?" is probably the most common question men newly diagnosed with prostate cancer ask their urologists. For now, there are no definitive answers about whether food choices can affect the recurrence of prostate disease. Meanwhile, a clinical trial published in 2020 found no evidence that a diet

Secondary prevention

Chan JM, Van Blarigan EL, Kenfield SA. What Should We Tell Prostate Cancer Patients About (Secondary) Prevention? *Current Opinion in Urology* 2014;24(3):318–23. PMID: 24625429.

PubMed See page 120.

rich in fruits, vegetables, whole grains, and legumes slows prostate cancer progression in men on active surveillance. (For reference, see "Diet, exercise, and weight loss," at left.) Still, we do know that prostate cancer, especially in its more aggressive forms, is more common in countries where men eat a Western diet containing relatively large amounts of meat. And studies suggest that good nutrition, including at least five servings a day of fruits and vegetables, improves the chances of surviving cancer in general.

Exercise

Regular exercise pares down your risk of developing some deadly problems, including heart disease, stroke, and certain types of cancer. And although relatively few studies have directly assessed the impact of exercise on prostate health, those that have been done have suggested that men who are more physically active are less likely to suffer from BPH or erectile dysfunction. Other studies have found that men with prostate cancer who engaged in vigorous exercise at least three hours a week were less likely to have their cancer progress or were less likely to die from the illness. For a study published in 2021, investigators split 52 men on active surveillance for prostate cancer (average age 63 and risk level ranging from very low-risk to favorable intermediate-risk) into two groups. One group underwent 12 weeks of high-intensity interval training three times a week, and the other group did not. Not surprisingly, the exercise regimen increased cardiorespiratory fitness, as measured by peak oxygen consumption. But in addition, prostate-specific antigen (PSA) levels either decreased among men in the exercise group, or increased at a slower rate. The results are encouraging, but larger studies are needed to determine if these improvements translate into long-term health benefits. (For references, see "Diet, exercise, and weight loss," at left.)

Guidelines from the American College of Sports Medicine recommend that cancer patients start exercising as soon as possible after or even during treatment. Exercising regularly can improve your physical state, helping you regain strength and conditioning you might have lost during cancer treatment. It reduces depression and fatigue and improves self-esteem. Combined with a healthy diet, exercise can also help to boost metabolic health in men undergoing hormonal therapy. The particular type of activity you choose is less important than finding one that you like, because you're more likely to stick with an activity you enjoy. The standard advice is to get at least a half-hour of physical activity on all or most days of the week. But any activity is better than none.

Weight loss

Evidence is accumulating that losing extra pounds, or avoiding weight gain in the first place, might help keep a prostate tumor in check. It is not yet clear why obesity might worsen outcomes of prostate cancer. Some research suggests that men who are obese tend to have lower PSA levels than those of normal weight. As a result, obese men may not be diagnosed until their cancers start growing aggressively. Other research indicates that excess fat in a person's body may increase levels of hormones that fuel tumor growth. (For references, see "Diet, exercise, and weight loss," at left.)

Diet, exercise, and weight loss

Freedland SJ, Howard L, Allen J, et al. A Lifestyle Intervention of Weight Loss via a Low-Carbohydrate Diet Plus Walking to Reduce Metabolic Disturbances Caused by Androgen Deprivation Therapy Among Prostate Cancer Patients: Carbohydrate and Prostate Study 1 (CAPS1) Randomized Controlled Trial. *Prostate Cancer and Prostatic Diseases* 2019;22(3):428–27. PMID: 30664736.

Kang DW, Fairey AS, Boulé NG, et al. Effects of Exercise on Cardiorespiratory Fitness and Biochemical Progression in Men with Localized Prostate Cancer Under Active Surveillance: The ERASE Randomized Clinical Trial. *JAMA Oncology* 2021;7(10):1487–95. PMID: 34410322.

Parsons JK, Zahrieh D, Mohler JL, et al. Effect of a Behavioral Intervention to Increase Vegetable Consumption on Cancer Progression Among Men with Early-Stage Prostate Cancer: The MEAL Randomized Clinical Trial. *JAMA* 2020;323(2):140–8. PMID: 31935026.

Troeschel AN, Hartman TJ, Jacobs EJ, et al. Postdiagnosis Body Mass Index, Weight Change, and Mortality from Prostate Cancer, Cardiovascular Disease, and All Causes Among Survivors of Nonmetastatic Prostate Cancer. *Journal of Clinical Oncology* 2020;38(18):2018–27. PMID: 32250715.

Wang Y, Jacobs EJ, Gapstur SM, et al. Recreational Physical Activity in Relation to Prostate Cancer–Specific Mortality Among Men with Nonmetastatic Prostate Cancer. *European Urology* 2017;72(6):931–9. PMID: 28711382.

Zuniqa KB, Chan JM, Ryan CJ, et al. Diet and Lifestyle Considerations for Patients with Prostate Cancer. *Urologic Oncology* 2020;38(3):105–17. PMID: 31327752.

Smoking cessation

If you're a smoker looking for another reason to quit, consider this: in addition to raising your risk of heart and lung disease, smoking could boost the odds that you will develop aggressive prostate cancer that metastasizes. Pooling data from 51 studies involving four million men, researchers found that smokers have a 24% higher risk of death from prostate cancer than nonsmokers. In a 2018 study of men treated for prostate cancer and followed for an average of six years after treatment, smokers were nearly twice as likely to die of their disease (89% higher risk) than nonsmokers. In addition, the risk that their cancers would spread was 151% higher, and there was a 40% higher risk that their PSA levels would rise again after surgery, signaling the cancer's return. (For references, see "Smoking and prostate cancer," at right.)

Use herbs and supplements with care—or not at all

About one-third (and maybe more) of American men with prostate cancer use at least one form of herbal or "natural" remedy—and that figure doesn't include men who use acupuncture, massage, or another complementary therapy.

Some herbs and supplements can interact with each other or with prescribed medications. Herbs can enhance the effects of medications or sometimes negate any benefit. One of the most common interactions involves herbs that affect the liver by acting on cytochrome P450 enzymes, which metabolize drugs. Many herbs, such as St. John's wort, have this effect. Others, like saw palmetto, which some men take for BPH, and melatonin, which some men take hoping it will slow the progression of prostate cancer, may increase the risk of bleeding when taken with aspirin, ibuprofen, naproxen, anticoagulants, or antiplatelet medications. In some cases, supplements have proved to be dangerous. That's why it's important to be open with your doctors and tell them if you're taking herbs or vitamins or pursuing some other form of non-traditional therapy.

Few large, high-quality clinical trials have assessed herbal remedies or supplements—and when they do, surprises sometimes emerge. The SELECT study, which tested whether vitamin E or selenium might affect prostate cancer risk, is a case in point. On the basis of earlier studies, researchers thought that vitamin E supplements might reduce the risk of prostate cancer. Instead, the SELECT study has consistently shown they are associated with a higher risk for prostate cancer. (For references, see "SELECT study," at right.)

Similarly, vitamin D has been shown to reduce the amounts of testosterone and dihydrotestosterone in blood and inhibit the growth of hormone-sensitive prostate cancer cells in the lab. But the evidence that vitamin D might protect against prostate cancer or even play a role in treating the disease is controversial. A review of 22 studies published in 2018 found no convincing evidence of a benefit from vitamin D supplements in terms of lowering prostate cancer risk. (For reference, see "Vitamin D," at right.)

Smoking and prostate cancer

Foerster B, Pozo C, Abufaraj M, et al. Association of Smoking Status with Recurrence, Metastasis and Mortality Among Patients with Localized Prostate Cancer Undergoing Prostatectomy or Radiotherapy: A Systematic Review and Meta-Analysis. *JAMA Oncology* 2018;4(7): 953–61. PMID: 29800115.

Islami F, Moreira DM, Boffetta P, et al. A Systematic Review and Meta-Analysis of Tobacco Use and Prostate Cancer Mortality and Incidence in Prospective Cohort Studies. *European Urology* 2014;66(6):1054–64. PMID: 25242554.

Riviere P, Kumar A, Luterstein E, et al. Tobacco Smoking and Death from Prostate Cancer in US Veterans. *Prostate Cancer and Prostatic Diseases* 2020;23(2):252–59. PMID: 31624316.

SELECT study

Klein EA, Thompson IM Jr, Tangen CM, et al. Vitamin E and the Risk of Prostate Cancer: The Selenium and Vitamin E Cancer Prevention Trial (SELECT). *JAMA* 2011;306(14):1549–56. PMID: 21990298.

Kristal AR, Darke AK, Morris JS, et al. Baseline Selenium Status and Effects of Selenium and Vitamin E Supplementation on Prostate Cancer Risk. *Journal of the National Cancer Institute* 2014;106(3):djt456. PMID: 24563519.

Vitamin D

Shahvazi S, Soltani S, Ahmadi SM, et al. The Effect of Vitamin D Supplementation on Prostate Cancer: A Systematic Review and Meta-Analysis of Clinical Trials. *Hormone and Metabolic Research* 2018;51(1):11–21. PMID: 30522147.

PubMed See page 120.

Searching PubMed in five easy steps

You can find and read the studies that are referenced in the pages of this report by searching PubMed, a resource of the National Library of Medicine. You can read abstracts (short summaries) of the studies for free, but in some cases you will have to pay to obtain the full report.

Here's how to access an abstract:

1. Open up your browser's window while connected to the Internet. Type www.pubmed.gov in the address bar and hit return.
2. This brings you to the PubMed welcome page. You will see the following:

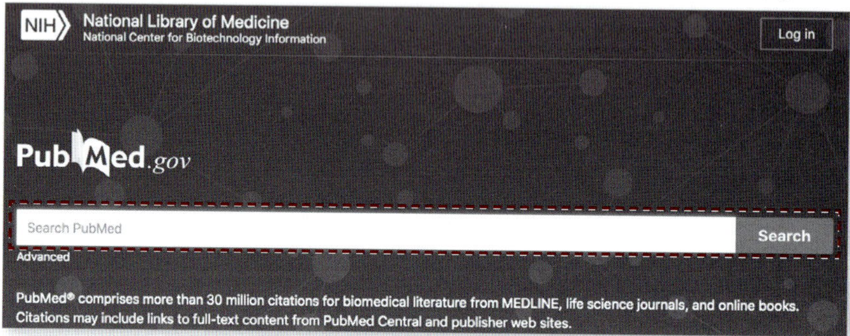

3. In the search box at the top of the page, type the PMID (short for "PubMed ID") number that appears with the reference you want. For example, for the study by Nicolosi et al., published in 2019 in *JAMA Oncology* (see "Genes and prostate cancer," page 39), the PMID is 30730552.

4. Click on "Search" or press the enter key. PubMed will retrieve the abstract, which will appear on your screen.
5. If the journal provides a link for purchase—or if a link is provided for a free copy of the article—click on the icon and follow the instructions.

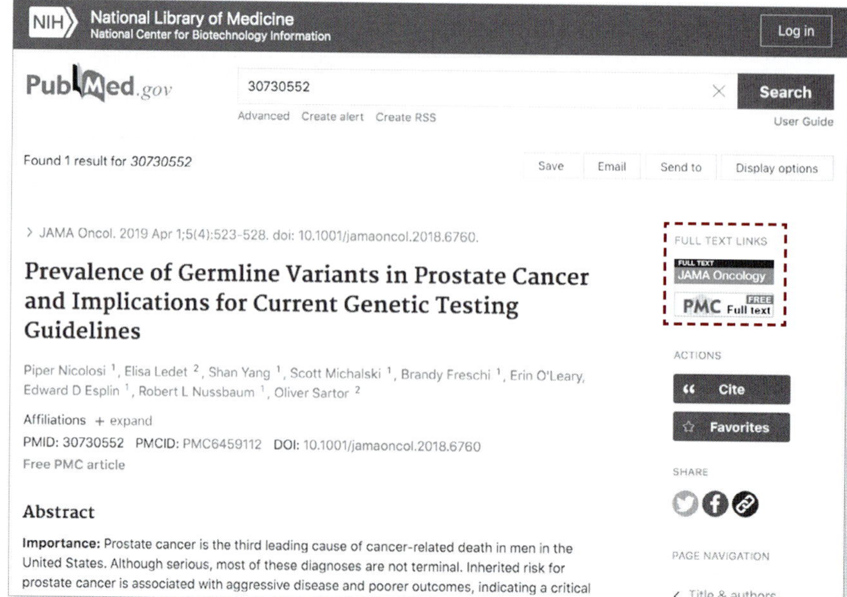

Information in this report is updated periodically online.

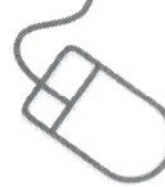

To access updated content at your convenience, visit www.health.harvard.edu/topics/prostate-health.

Resources

American Urological Association (AUA)
1000 Corporate Blvd.
Linthicum, MD 21090
410-689-3700
www.auanet.org

The AUA is a professional association for the advancement of urologic patient care. It helps physicians and patients stay current on the latest research and practices in urology. The AUA also provides a range of services, including publications, research, meetings, and guidance on health policy.

Harvard Health Publishing (HHP)
Harvard Medical School
4 Blackfan Circle, 4th floor
Boston, MA 02115
877-649-9457 (toll-free)
www.health.harvard.edu
www.health.harvard.edu/topics/prostate-health

A division of Harvard Medical School, HHP publishes subscription newsletters, in-depth health reports on a variety of topics and medical conditions, and books. HHP also maintains a section on its website dedicated to prostate health. It includes articles on prostate diseases from the company's publications as well as brief summaries of groundbreaking prostate research. Experiences of individual patients with various prostate problems are summarized in the Special Health Report *Patient Perspectives on Prostate Diseases.*

National Cancer Institute (NCI)
Office of Communications and Public Liaison
9609 Medical Center Drive, MSC 9760
Bethesda, MD 20892
800-422-6237 (toll-free)
www.cancer.gov
www.cancercontrol.cancer.gov/ocs

This government agency, part of the National Institutes of Health, conducts and sponsors research on all types of cancer. Operators can answer questions, provide informational booklets and brochures on prostate cancer, and make referrals to local resources. The NCI also offers the latest information about cancer clinical trials, including their locations. The website provides online information for patients, health professionals, and the public.

Prostate Cancer Foundation
1250 Fourth St.
Santa Monica, CA 90401
800-757-2873 (toll-free)
www.pcf.org

This philanthropic organization funds prostate cancer research. Its website offers general information about prostate cancer; a list of resources for patients needing financial assistance; help finding a doctor or treatment center; and support for patients, families, and caregivers.

Zero—The End of Prostate Cancer
515 King St., Suite 420
Alexandria, VA 22314
202-463-9455
https://zerocancer.org

This nonprofit provides a comprehensive range of services for people with prostate cancer, including information on prostate cancer and treatment, support groups (both in-person and online), a physician finder, and financial assistance for people in a number of states to help pay for transportation to and from appointments. To find the chapter nearest you, visit the website.

Glossary

abscopal effect: A byproduct of cancer treatment in which radiation or other types of localized therapy shrink not only the targeted tumor, but also untreated tumors elsewhere in the body.

active surveillance: A strategy for managing prostate cancer in which the patient is regularly examined but is not treated until the disease shows signs of worsening.

acute urinary retention: An inability to squeeze any urine past an enlarged prostate because the bladder has become distended and its muscular wall has weakened.

adjuvant radiation: Radiation given shortly after initial surgery for cancer as an additional (adjuvant) treatment, when there is a presumption of residual cancer—even without a rise in PSA levels or signs of cancer on a scan.

alpha blocker: A type of medication used to treat high blood pressure, benign prostatic hyperplasia, and chronic prostatitis.

androgen deprivation therapy (ADT): See hormonal therapy.

androgens: The male hormones, particularly testosterone and dihydrotestosterone (DHT).

anti-androgens: Drugs used in hormonal therapy that work by inhibiting the dihydrotestosterone (DHT) in prostate cells.

antimuscarinics: Drugs that block receptors in the smooth muscle tissue in the bladder wall so that this muscle is less likely to contract.

aquablation: A robot-assisted surgical technique that destroys prostate tissue with jets of highly pressurized salt solution.

AR-V7: A gene mutation that helps to predict if a man's prostate cancer will respond to the hormonal therapies abiraterone (Zytiga) or enzalutamide (Xtandi).

benign prostatic hyperplasia (BPH): A noncancerous enlargement of the prostate that can cause problems with urination.

biochemical recurrence: A post-treatment increase in PSA level, indicating that prostate cancer has recurred or spread following the original treatment for prostate cancer.

biomarker: A distinctive biological indicator of an event, process, or condition.

biopsy: A procedure in which small samples of tissue are removed for analysis under a microscope.

brachytherapy: A form of radiation treatment using seeds or pellets of radioactive material, which are implanted in the prostate to destroy cancer cells.

BRCA1, BRCA2: Two tumor suppressor genes that, when mutated, increase the risk for breast and ovarian cancers in women and aggressive prostate cancer in men.

catheter: A narrow, flexible tube inserted into the urethra and up into the bladder to allow passage of urine when someone is unable to urinate.

checkpoint inhibitor: A type of drug that blocks cellular checkpoints, which are proteins that cancer cells use to shield themselves from the immune system. Checkpoint inhibitors intensify the immune system's attack on cancer.

chemotherapy: The use of specific medications to eradicate cancer cells.

circulating tumor cells: Cells that are shed by tumors into the bloodstream that may seed new tumors elsewhere in the body.

circulating tumor DNA: DNA released into the bloodstream by tumor cells.

computed tomography (CT): An imaging method that combines x-ray images taken from different angles and uses computer processing to create cross-sectional views of the bones, blood vessels, and soft tissues.

core: A piece of tissue obtained in a biopsy of the prostate.

cryotherapy: A surgical procedure that eliminates abnormal tissue by freezing it.

de novo metastatic cancer: Newly diagnosed metastatic cancer in someone who has not yet been treated for the disease.

digital rectal examination (DRE): A screening test in which the physician inserts a gloved finger into the rectum to examine the prostate for abnormalities.

endorectal coil MRI: Magnetic resonance imaging done with a coil (consisting of a probe and an inflatable balloon) inserted into the rectum. The test helps doctors assess cancer spread and local invasion.

erectile dysfunction (ED): A more specific term for impotence that refers to the inability to have and maintain an erection sufficient for intercourse.

Glossary *continued*

false negative: A test result that indicates a person does not have a disease or condition when the person actually does have it.

false positive: A test result that indicates a person has a disease or condition that the person actually does not have.

5-alpha-reductase inhibitors: A class of drugs used to help shrink the prostate as a treatment for benign prostatic hyperplasia. They block the action of the enzyme 5-alpha reductase, which converts testosterone to dihydrotestosterone (DHT). The latter stimulates prostate growth.

focal therapy: Treatment intended to remove or destroy only the cancerous portion of the prostate and to spare healthy prostate tissue.

free PSA: PSA circulating in the blood that is not bound to other proteins.

germline mutations: Mutations in sperm or egg cells that can be passed down to newly formed embryos. Such mutations exist in all cells of the body.

Gleason score: A numerical grade that describes prostate cancer based on its aggressiveness.

GnRH antagonists: Gonadotropin-releasing hormone antagonists. Like LHRH agonists, these drugs treat prostate cancer by blocking the release of luteinizing hormone (LH), but without a temporary surge in testosterone.

high-intensity focused ultrasound (HIFU): A treatment that ablates, or destroys, tumors with heat generated by ultrasound energy.

high-volume cancer: A term used to describe a tumor that occupies a large amount of the prostate gland.

hormonal therapy: Treatment for prostate cancer (with either drugs or, in rare cases, surgery) that is intended to reduce or eliminate the supply of male hormones to the prostate and distant cancer sites, thereby slowing cancer growth. Also referred to as androgen deprivation therapy (ADT).

HOXC6/DLX1: A genetic biomarker that predicts high-grade prostate cancer in men flagged by PSA screening.

immuno-oncology: The study and development of treatments that harness the immune system to fight cancer.

immunotherapy: Treatments designed to turn the body's immune system against cancer in the body.

impotence: See erectile dysfunction.

indolent: A term that describes slow-growing tumors that will ordinarily not cause symptoms or be life-threatening.

intensity-modulated radiation therapy (IMRT): High-precision delivery of radiation in multiple beams adjusted to conform to the three-dimensional shape of a tumor.

laparoscopy: A surgical approach in which a procedure is carried out with tiny instruments inserted through small openings in the skin.

LHRH agonists: Drugs used to treat prostate cancer by blocking chemical messages that signal the body's cells to make testosterone.

localized: A term used to describe cancer that is limited to a specific gland, organ, or other tissue, without any distant spread.

luteinizing hormone (LH): A hormone released from the brain that controls the production of androgens by the testes.

lymph nodes: Small, specialized clusters of tissue that help fight infections and capture cancer cells that have moved out of a given tissue or organ.

magnetic resonance imaging (MRI): A test that relies on magnetic fields to visualize abnormalities in the body.

medical oncologist: A physician who specializes in chemotherapy, hormonal therapy, biological therapy, and targeted therapy for cancer; usually the main health care provider for someone with cancer.

metastasis: The spread of cancer throughout the body, beyond the organ or tissue in which it originated.

metastasis-directed therapy: The use of radiation, surgery, and other treatments targeted specifically at metastatic tumors.

metastatic castration-resistant prostate cancer (mCRPC): Metastatic cancer that doesn't respond to hormonal therapy.

metastatic castration-sensitive prostate cancer (mCSPC): Metastatic cancer that responds to hormonal therapy.

mismatch repair genes: Genes that help to repair DNA damage. Alterations in these genes can allow cancers to develop.

MyProstateScore (MPS): A genetic test for prostate cancer that measures PSA, PCA3, and TMPRSS2:ERG in urine.

Glossary *continued*

multiparametric MRI: A hybrid imaging technique that combines several different MRI strategies to improve diagnostic accuracy.

nanograms per milliliter (ng/ml): A small quantity of a substance equivalent to one-billionth of a gram (454 grams make 1 pound) in one-thousandth of a liter (1 liter is approximately 1 quart).

nerve-sparing prostatectomy: A surgical procedure for prostate removal, designed to avoid damaging the nerves that are necessary for potency.

nonmetastatic castration-resistant prostate cancer (nmCRPC): A condition marked by rising PSA levels after initial prostate cancer treatment, without visible metastases, that persists despite the use of hormonal therapy.

nonmetastatic castration-sensitive prostate cancer (nmCSPC): A condition marked by rising PSA levels after initial prostate cancer treatment, without visible metastases, that responds to hormonal therapy.

oligometastatic prostate cancer: Cancer with five or fewer detectable metastases detected on imaging scans.

oligoprogressive prostate cancer: Oligometastatic cancer that continues to grow.

oncologist: A physician who deals with the diagnosis and treatment of cancer. There are three types of oncologists—medical oncologists, radiation oncologists, and surgical oncologists.

open prostatectomy: A surgical procedure in which prostate tissue is removed through an incision in the abdomen.

PARP inhibitor: A drug used for treating men with BRCA-positive prostate cancer.

PCA3: A genetic prostate cancer biomarker found in urine.

PDE5 inhibitors: Drugs that block PDE5, an enzyme that breaks down erection-producing chemicals. These drugs can help a man achieve and maintain an erection.

perineum: The area between the anus and the scrotum (in males) or the anus and vulva (in females).

photoselective vaporization of the prostate (PVP): A procedure for treating benign prostatic hyperplasia that uses laser light to vaporize excess prostate tissue.

placebo: A pill with no active ingredients or a sham procedure, used in studies to provide a basis of comparison with an active treatment.

positron emission tomography (PET): An imaging approach that measures metabolic activity in cells.

priapism: A potentially painful medical condition in which the erect penis does not return to its flaccid state.

primary cancer: The original cancer in the prostate, from which metastatic disease originates.

prostate-specific antigen (PSA): A protein produced by the prostate. Elevated PSA levels may indicate the presence of cancer, benign prostatic hyperplasia, or prostatitis. A PSA test measures the level of this protein in the blood.

prostate-specific membrane antigen (PSMA): A protein found at high levels on the surface of prostate cancer cells.

prostatic artery embolization: A nonsurgical technique for treating benign prostatic hyperplasia. The procedure involves the insertion of tiny particles into the artery that serves the prostate, thus blocking blood flow, which in turn causes prostate tissues to shrink.

prostatic urethral lift: A minimally invasive procedure for treating benign prostatic hyperplasia that uses clamps and sutures to lift the prostate and hold it away from the urethra, thereby allowing urine to flow more freely.

prostatic urethral stent: A small, springlike cylinder designed to relieve pressure from prostatic tissue and improve urine flow. It is positioned in the narrowed area of the urethra and released to widen the channel.

prostatitis: Inflammation or infection of the prostate that may result in painful or difficult urination.

PSA velocity: The rate at which a man's PSA level increases over time.

PTEN: A tumor suppressor gene that, if defective, may allow prostate cancer to develop.

radiation oncologist: A physician who specializes in the use of radiation to treat cancer.

radiation therapy: Treatment with high-energy rays (from x-rays or other sources) designed to destroy cancer cells.

radiation toxicity: Damage to tissues resulting from radiation treatment to the prostate and surrounding areas; can include inflammation and damage to the lower parts of the colon.

radical prostatectomy: A surgical procedure used to remove the prostate, seminal vesicles, and pelvic lymph nodes.

Glossary *continued*

radiofrequency ablation: A type of therapy that uses electrical energy and heat to destroy cancerous tissues.

resectoscope: An instrument that permits a surgeon to view the prostate during transurethral resection.

retrograde ejaculation: A side effect of prostate surgery and some medications, in which semen flows back into the bladder rather than out through the penis.

Rezum: See water vapor thermal therapy.

risk factor: A characteristic or feature that predisposes an individual to develop a certain type of cancer or other disease; a feature whose presence may affect prognosis.

salvage radiation: Radiation given to treat suspected recurrent cancer; in the case of prostate cancer, it is given in response to rising PSA levels after initial surgery.

seminal vesicles: Structures next to the prostate gland that produce seminal fluid.

somatic mutations: Mutations that develop in DNA in cells other than sperm or egg cells as a result of aging or environmental exposures or sometimes for no clear reason. They are not inherited.

stereotactic body radiation therapy (SBRT): A procedure that delivers high doses of radiation to tumor sites throughout the body, usually in soft tissues, with guidance from imaging; also called stereotactic ablative radiation therapy.

surgical margin: An edge of normal-looking tissue surrounding an excised tumor. The margins can be checked for cancer under a microscope after the tumor is removed.

surgical oncologist: A physician specializing in surgery for cancer.

systemic treatment: Hormonal therapies, chemotherapy, or targeted therapies used for treating cancer throughout the body.

targeted therapy: Drugs or other agents that attack cancer cells containing specific genetic mutations.

TMPRSS2:ERG gene fusion: A fusion of two genes that is present in roughly half of all prostate cancers and detectable in urine.

transperineal biopsy: A method to access the prostate with a biopsy needle inserted through the perineum.

transrectal ultrasonography: A procedure that uses sound waves to create an image of the prostate. The sound waves are generated from a probe inserted in the rectum.

transrectal ultrasound-guided (TRUS) biopsy: A method of taking samples from the prostate through the rectum under ultrasound guidance. Also called a standard biopsy.

transurethral electrovaporization of the prostate (TUEVP or TVP): A procedure used to treat benign prostatic hyperplasia that uses electrical energy to heat, vaporize, and cauterize prostate tissue.

transurethral incision of the prostate (TUIP): An operation used to treat benign prostatic hyperplasia in which incisions are made in the prostate tissue to relieve pressure on the urethra and alleviate urinary difficulties.

transurethral microwave thermotherapy (TUMT): A heat therapy for benign prostatic hyperplasia that uses microwaves to destroy prostate tissue that obstructs urine flow.

transurethral needle ablation (TUNA): A procedure used to treat benign prostatic hyperplasia that uses radio waves to heat and destroy prostate cells obstructing the urethra.

transurethral resection of the prostate (TURP): The most common procedure to treat benign prostatic hyperplasia, in which excess prostate tissue is cut away.

urethra: The tube that transports urine from the bladder (and semen from the prostate and seminal vesicles) out through the penis.

urinary incontinence: The inability to control urine flow, resulting in involuntary discharge or leakage.

urologist: A physician who deals with the urinary tract and male reproductive system.

vasectomy: An operation that cuts and seals the tubes through which sperm cells travel from the testicles so they can mix with semen. A man continues to ejaculate, but the semen doesn't contain sperm.

water vapor thermal therapy: A procedure that uses steam to shrink an enlarged prostate. Frequently referred to by the brand name Rezum.

Notes

Notes

Notes